Practical
Nursing

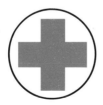

British Red Cross Society
in association with
Dorling Kindersley Limited London

First edition published in Great Britain in 1984 by
Dorling Kindersley Limited, 9 Henrietta Street
Covent Garden, London WC2 8PS
Reprinted 1984, 1985, 1990

British Library Cataloguing in Publication Data
Practical Nursing
    1. Home nursing
    I. Red Cross. *British Red Cross Society*
    649.8   RT61

ISBN 0–86318–137–X

Contents

Introduction	**5**	**Daily routines**	**46**
		Taking a temperature	47
Preparing for a patient	**6**	Pulse	48
Cleanliness	8	Breathing	49
Adapting a room	8	Giving medicines	49
		Medicines by mouth	50
Preparing for a new baby	**9**	Inhalation	51
Selecting equipment	9	Food and diet	52
The baby's room	10	A balanced diet	52
		Dietary essentials	54
The patient in bed	**12**	Food presentation	56
Bedding	13	Special diets	57
Bedmaking	14	Feeding a baby	58
When a patient cannot get up	16	Breast-feeding	59
Drawsheets	17	Bottle-feeding	60
Moving a patient	18		
Moving a patient up a high bed	18	**Injuries**	**62**
Moving a patient up a low bed	19	Caring for wounds	64
Turning a patient in bed	20	Roller bandages	66
Moving a patient from bed to chair	21	Applying an arm sling	68
Moving a patient alone	22	Reef knots	68
Comfort in bed	24	Inflammation	70
Extra warmth	25		
Positions for bedrest	26	**Infectious diseases**	**72**
Pressure areas	27	Nursing care	74
		Containing infection	75
Personal care	**28**		
The bathroom	29	**Special nursing**	**76**
Giving a bed bath	30	The patient home from hospital	77
Hair care	31	Nursing the elderly	78
Caring for nails	31	Handicapped children	80
Care of the mouth	32	Physical handicaps	80
Bathing a baby	33	Mental handicaps	82
Clothes	34	Aids in nursing	83
Dressing and undressing	34	Aids to dressing	84
Baby clothes	36	Bathroom aids	85
Dressing a baby	36		
Elimination	38	**Preventing accidents**	**86**
Faeces	39	The entrance hall	87
Daily excretions	40	Kitchen safety	88
Incontinence	40	The living room	90
Nappies	42	Stairs and windows	92
Sterilising nappies	44		
Control of bowel and bladder	45	Index	94

Foreword

This book replaces the two manuals
Practical Infant and Child Care and
Practical Nursing first published in 1973
and 1976 respectively.

The work is the result of a team effort
co-ordinated by the Director of Marketing
Services of the British Red Cross Society,
Mr J. M. Jerram. The Director of Training,
Miss Margaret Baker BA MIHE has given
invaluable guidance on both presentation
and use as a teaching aid.

Our thanks are due to Miss Moyra M.
Heggie SRN HVcert NDN SCM MTD
Midwifery Tutor King's College Hospital,
London, and to Mrs B. Macleod SRN
HVcert. FWcert., Clinical Nurse Manager,
Kettering Health Authority, for updating
the sections Infant and Child Care.

Miss Edith R. Parker MSc BA(Hons)
SRN RMN SCM RNT, Branch Nursing
Advisor London Branch, Nurse Member of
Council and Director of Nurse Education,
The Princess Alexandra School of Nursing,
The London Hospital, Whitechapel,
London E1 has advised on current nursing
practice and spent a considerable amount
of time on proof reading and correction.

To Michael McGeorge JP SRN NDN
Nursing Officer National Headquarters
must go the credit for the major part of
this project in re-writing, updating and
collating the content of two manuals
resulting in one excellent book.

Finally, the Society acknowledges its
debt to the publishers, Dorling Kindersley,
who in this, as in other publications of the
Society, have brought a fresh approach in
presentation of our manuals.

Sheila Quinn CBE BSc(Econ) Hons SRN SCM
RNT FRCN FHA
Nursing Advisor to
The British Red Cross Society

Introduction

What is nursing? It is the skilled care of someone who is ill, injured or in any way physically or mentally handicapped. It involves looking after the basic physical needs of an individual whilst also having regard to his or her likes and requirements. The aim of nursing is for a patient to regain his or her health as speedily as possible.

Home nursing care

At some time in our lives most of us look after someone else at home. This might be someone who is ill and needs nursing care, a child who is handicapped, a new baby or an elderly person, for example. You need to know how best to help, doing for the person in your care what he or she cannot manage and encouraging an early return to full independence. The skills, methods, information and ideas in this book will give you the basic knowledge to look after someone at home.

Most home care is given by members of the family and this book is aimed at all age groups. It will be of particular use to young people who may be involved in caring for others for the first time. Any special treatments will be given by a district nurse or doctor who will include you as a welcome member of the health team if you show the qualities of a good nurse.

Relations with the patient

When you are looking after someone who is unwell, he or she may be frightened by the illness, worried or in pain. Be comforting and show confident practical ability so that the patient and family can trust you.

Explain what is happening in any nursing procedures, what is required of the patient and how you will help. Do not be in a hurry. You may need to reassure the patient or repeat an explanation. Be tolerant when a patient is difficult to help or is slow to perform everyday tasks. Remember that your company and willingness to provide a listening ear may be very valuable to anyone who is lonely or anxious. Show your sympathy, never let yourself get irritated with a patient but be quietly firm about any medical instructions you have been asked to carry out. Your movements should be gentle and calm. Your friendly care is important whether or not a patient can respond; a stroke patient, for example, may be unable to speak but will be aware of your mood and your concern for his or her welfare.

Character and appearance

Reliability is essential when you are nursing. Carry out instructions punctually and exactly as given. Be discreet and observant. Watch the patient's progress so that you can report any change to the nurse or doctor, but do not alarm the patient by your observations and do not discuss his or her condition with anyone other than the medical team.

Be clean and tidy, both in your person and in the way you work. Do not wear jewellery or a wrist watch when handling a patient because it might cause a skin injury.

About this book

Those pages with information about caring for babies are identified by a yellow tint to make them easy to pick out. Some material, such as the chapter on preventing accidents whilst not strictly speaking nursing, is included because of its practical relevance.

Preparing for a patient

Patients cannot always choose their surroundings and so may be dependent on your forethought. Try to provide a calm and happy atmosphere. Think about what you can do to make the room comfortable for the patient as well as practical for you to nurse in. Your attitude and that of the family and friends can help by being caring and unhurried. Do not ever let the patient feel a burden.

The patient's room

Most people prefer to be looked after in their own bedroom. You may need to reorganise a room to make it practical for nursing, but do take account of the patient's wishes so that the results are acceptable to him or her.

If possible, place the bed so that the patient can see out of the window particularly if there is an attractive outlook. If the room is overlooked, net curtains or blinds may be necessary to protect the patient's privacy. These are also useful in controlling the light.

A single bed with a firm but comfortable mattress is ideal because it will give support to the patient and allow easy access for nursing. However, if the patient must be cared for in a double bed and is sharing it, there is the considerable advantage of having someone close by at night.

A commode is necessary for patients who are able to get out of bed but are unable or unwilling to go as far as the lavatory. If the patient can get to the bathroom, make access as easy as possible by removing hazards which might be tripped over in the passageways. A carpet in the bedroom helps to reduce noise and is less slippery for someone who is unsteady.

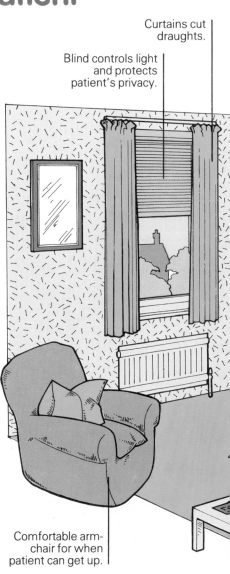

Curtains cut draughts.

Blind controls light and protects patient's privacy.

Comfortable armchair for when patient can get up.

Table offers a good work top for equipment. Protect the surface.

The chest serves as bedside table for things patient wants within reach and storage for belongings.

Adequate shelf space makes it easy to keep sickroom tidy.

Single bed allows clear access on three sides.

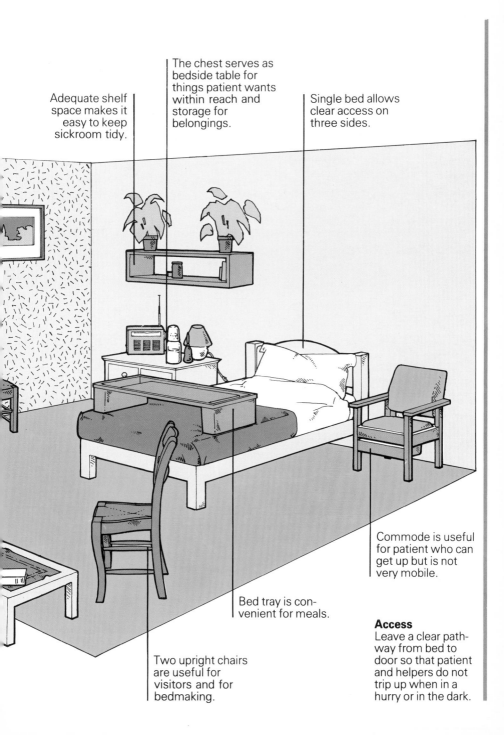

Commode is useful for patient who can get up but is not very mobile.

Bed tray is convenient for meals.

Two upright chairs are useful for visitors and for bedmaking.

Access
Leave a clear pathway from bed to door so that patient and helpers do not trip up when in a hurry or in the dark.

Cleanliness

Good hygiene is essential. Bacteria can spread from person to person and dust settling on a wound or food can also be a source of infection to the patient. Clean the room thoroughly without raising dust, using a damp mop and a carpet sweeper or vacuum cleaner. The room should be free of unpleasant smells, well ventilated and comfortably warm. After a commode or bedpan has been used or after meals, use a fresh air spray if there is an odour left in the room. Empty and wipe out the waste-paper bin each day. Fresh air is important but the patient should not be in a draught. If it is too hot he or she may sweat uncomfortably and if it is too cool may catch a chill.

Adapting a room

Patients should be looked after in their own room if possible. You may have to move someone to another room for various reasons, but do this only in the patient's interests, not simply for your own convenience. A move may be necessary for these reasons:
● to be nearer or on the same level as the bathroom
● when the bedroom cannot be used for the duration of illness — for example, if the patient normally shares a room with other children who should avoid contact with infection

● when another room provides a more comfortable and attractive environment than the patient's room
● when the patient's condition makes upstairs access impossible, perhaps due to confinement to a wheelchair.

Remember that the patient's needs remain the same as if being nursed in his or her own room. So even if the room is, say, a dining room which the whole family used to share, the need for privacy, quiet and an even temperature must be respected.

Hazards

For both your own and the patient's comfort and safety avoid the following unnecessary hazards in the bedroom:
● tall containers on the front of projecting surfaces can all too easily be knocked over by a helper in a hurry or an unsteady patient looking for support
● do not leave medicines by the bed — a dose could easily be repeated by mistake

● equipment left lying around which might trip you up
● elderly or sleepy patients should not be left alone while smoking in bed. Provide a large ashtray that will not tip over easily. If the patient is confused, be careful to remove matches and cigarettes from the bedside in case he or she sets the bed on fire. The patient's condition may make smoking unwise or even dangerous.

Preparing for a new baby

Young babies are extremely demanding. They cry when they are hungry or thirsty and for various other reasons. Discomfort from a wet or soiled nappy, wind, being too hot or cold may all produce a yell for attention. All babies need affection and constant care. Being loved and played with, cuddled and talked to are essential to a baby's development and sense of security.

Parents sometimes want very new babies to sleep in their bedroom at night. After the first few days, the parents will get more rest if the baby can be moved into his or her own bedroom. Of course they must be able to hear the baby crying but do not need to hear every snuffle.

Selecting equipment

A baby grows very rapidly during the first year of life and requires a great deal of sleep. The cot is the most important piece of furniture which is needed. A carry-cot will probably be the most practical sort for the first months. It can be carried everywhere and the baby can sleep in it day and night. Many carry-cots have a wheeled stand and a waterproof hood and cover so they can double as a pram. A straw Moses basket with handles is less adaptable, but is light and quite adequate for indoors. If a carry-cot is used in a car, it should be strapped down so that it will not be thrown off the seat in an accident. A small cot or cradle is comfortable and convenient for the baby, but it will be quickly outgrown so it is not practical if the budget is tight.

Bedtime
By the time the baby is six months or so, he or she will be needing a full-sized cot. The drop-sided wooden kind is probably the safest and most hard-wearing. Make sure that the side-lowering mechanism is strong but easy to work and that the bars are no more than 7cm (3in) apart or the baby's head could get stuck through them in a dangerous and uncomfortable position.

The mattress should be firm and preferably covered in a waterproof material which is easy to clean. It should fit the cot exactly so that the baby cannot get caught between cot sides and mattress. It should be thick enough to keep the baby warm and have a waterproof cover, which will need sponging down regularly. If a mattress is supplied in a plastic bag, dispose of the bag safely.

Bathtime
While the baby is very small, it is easier to keep a baby bath in the bedroom. They are often made of sloped rigid plastic and some designs are supplied with a collapsible stand (make sure it is really steady enough).

Sitting up
A high chair with a broad, steady base and safety straps will be useful. Its tray should be quite big with smooth corners for easy cleaning. Indeed, rounded corners are advisable on all children's furniture. A light baby-bouncer is also a good idea.

The baby's room

The room should be well ventilated but warm. Fresh air is important but protect babies from draughts and from chilling at night if the heating goes off. Central heating, oil-filled electric radiators and night-storage heaters are the safest forms of heating, oil heaters the most dangerous, causing innumerable fire deaths each year. Consider if the windows will be safe in a year or so when your baby becomes an enquiring and mobile toddler.

Decorating

Lead-free spongeable paint and vinyl wallpapers are easily cleaned of the grubby fingermarks which are likely to appear when the baby is more mobile. Light cheerful colours are stimulating. Wooden floors can be dangerous because of splinters when a child is crawling. Some synthetic carpets are soft and warm to the knees and easy to keep clean. Cork tiles and lino are also easy to clean. Any rugs should have a non-slip backing.

Switches and trailing flexes should be out of reach of prying fingers and put plugs into sockets even if they are not being used. Otherwise a child might insert something. The light will need to be adequate for baby care and later for the growing child to play by.

Small babies need only simple toys like rattles or soft furry animals to amuse them. Interesting pictures on the walls and mobiles suspended over the cot or from the ceiling will keep them happy too. By the time the baby is crawling, a playpen may be necessary to keep him or her in a safe environment for short periods while you are busy. Always provide some favourite toys in the playpen.

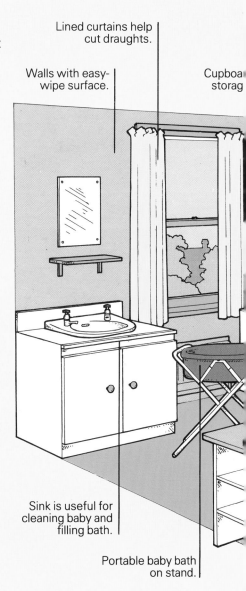

Lined curtains help cut draughts.

Walls with easy-wipe surface.

Cupboa storag

Sink is useful for cleaning baby and filling bath.

Portable baby bath on stand.

Flat surface fo changing. Storag below for nappie: baby lotion an cleaning equipmen

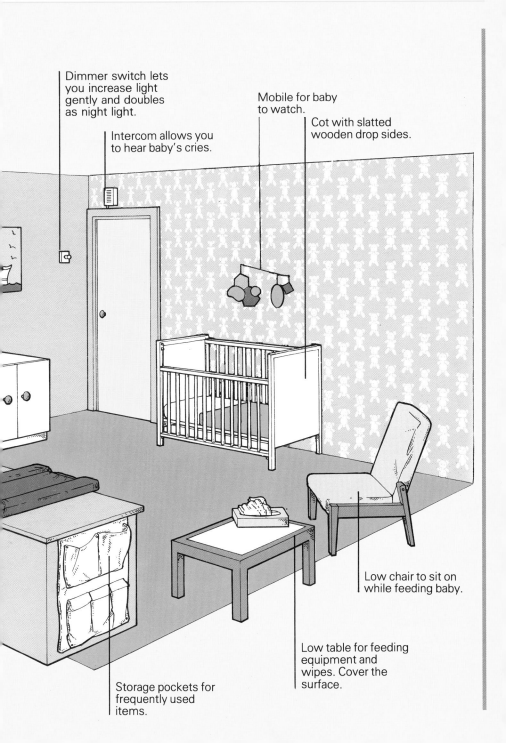

Dimmer switch lets you increase light gently and doubles as night light.

Intercom allows you to hear baby's cries.

Mobile for baby to watch.

Cot with slatted wooden drop sides.

Low chair to sit on while feeding baby.

Low table for feeding equipment and wipes. Cover the surface.

Storage pockets for frequently used items.

The patient in bed

Someone who is ill usually has to spend so much of their day in bed or getting in and out, that making the bed comfortable is one of the most important things you can do to help. If he or she is in bed all the time, the bedclothes should be straightened twice a day at least. The sheets will need changing every three days or so, more often if the patient is perspiring heavily.

Patients who are able to move around should be encouraged to do so as it helps their circulation. But be on hand if patients need help.

Prolonged bedrest brings its own problems. Patients confined to bed may risk circulatory problems with their legs and they are likely to develop pressure sores (see page 27). The doctor or district nursing sister/charge nurse will advise you on the gentle exercise which may be possible and patients should be turned in bed every couple of hours if they cannot move themselves unaided.

If the bed is quite low, as most home beds are, you should take care not to strain your back. When moving a bed or a patient always work with a helper if available. Knowing how best to lift and bend enables you to avoid unnecessary effort or injury (see pages 18–23).

Wooden bed blocks can be used to raise the foot of the bed (sometimes advisable for patients with swollen feet or legs) or the whole bed.

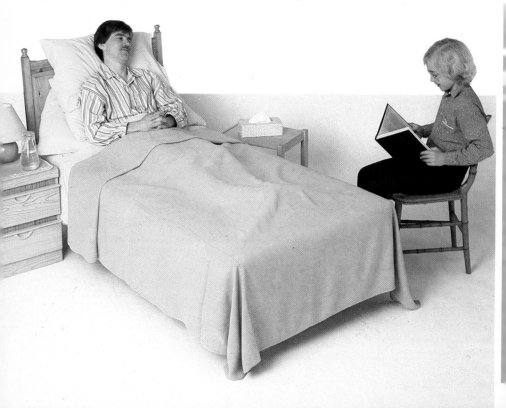

Bedding

Whether you make a bed with conventional sheets and blankets or a fitted sheet and duvet is a matter of personal preference. Consult the patient and try to use whatever he or she feels to be more comfortable. The techniques described in this section mostly apply to flat sheets and blankets because they are more complicated. However, the principles are exactly the same with a fitted sheet and duvet.

If blankets are used, cellular woollen ones are often preferred as they provide warmth without weight.

Duvets and fitted sheets

Continental quilts, or duvets, trap the air around the body, and form a warm light layer over the patient. They have separate washable covers and fillings of down, feather and down or man-made materials. Quilts with synthetic fillings may not be warm enough for all patients but can suit those prone to allergies. Duvets come in different sizes and should be at least 30cm (12in) wider than the bed. Do not use a bedspread as it will squash out the air and reduce the warmth. Duvets need to be shaken up regularly so that the filling remains evenly distributed, otherwise it will start to collect at the bottom. Bedmaking is quicker and simpler with a duvet but should not be done any less often because the patient will still want to come back to a freshly-made and aired bed after a bath or exercise.

Fitted sheets can be useful if you are nursing a very restless patient as they are less likely to ruck up. They do not usually need ironing because most are made from a cotton and synthetic mixture which creases little.

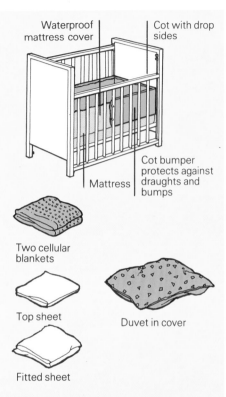

Waterproof mattress cover

Cot with drop sides

Mattress

Cot bumper protects against draughts and bumps

Two cellular blankets

Top sheet

Duvet in cover

Fitted sheet

Making a cot

This is quick and easy because cots are so small. Equipment varies, but to make the cot start by covering the mattress with a fitted quilted plastic (not polythene) sheet followed by a cotton or flannelette fitted undersheet. Put two blankets under the mattress, drawing the sides round over the baby to tuck in. Alternatively cover the baby with a washable continental quilt in a cover. Do not use pillows. A small baby could burrow into a pillow and suffocate. This amount of bedclothes will suit a well-wrapped up baby in a warm room.

Bedmaking

All the bedmaking methods are quicker and easier to carry out when there are two people to do them. So try to have a helper if possible. This chapter covers techniques for making a bed both with and without a patient in it. How you make a bed varies with the patient and what you have available. But there are some things which are standard.

You will need:
- an underblanket
- pillows (as many as necessary)
- two chairs back to back

and either
- two sheets
- two blankets
- an eiderdown for cold weather
- a bedspread

or
- a fitted sheet
- a duvet (continental quilt)
- a duvet cover.

Sometimes a plastic sheet may be needed to protect the mattress (if the bed is likely to become wet because a patient is incontinent). Plastic sheets and other special aids are available through the district nurse. If incontinence pads are used, they go under the buttocks above the bottom sheet. Drawsheets are occasionally useful when a patient perspires heavily and is unable to get up (see page 17).

Stripping a bed
When you strip a bed, have the two chairs back to back at the foot of the bed, ready for you to put the folded bedclothes on in the order you will want them to remake the bed. Put dirty linen in a bucket or large polythene bag. Fold the layers of bedclothes into three so that they are neat and do not touch the floor. Put the chairs back in position when you have made the bed.

Making mitred corners

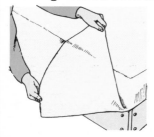

1 Tuck in the bottom sheet at the ends. Pick up the edges of the sheet about 45cm (18in) from the corner of the mattress. Tuck in the part of the sheet which hangs down.

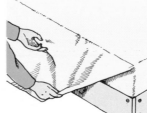

2 Bring down the fold of sheet you have been holding so that it hangs by the side of the bed.

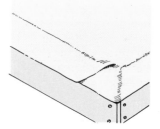

3 Tuck in the side of the sheet. Treat corners of the top sheet and blankets similarly at the bottom of the bed. They should be loosely tucked in so no pressure will be put on the feet.

Making an empty bed

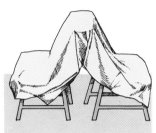
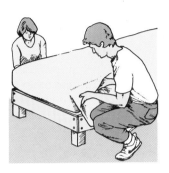
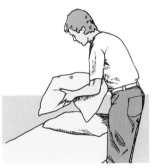

1 Put the bedclothes neatly on the two chairs at the end of the bed in the order you will need them. Cover the mattress with the under-blanket (put a plastic sheet under if needed).

2 Put the bottom sheet on with the right side up. If you are using a fitted sheet, ease the corners over the mattress. Otherwise tuck in the sheet making mitred corners.

3 Put the pillows on. *Either* put the top sheet in place wrong side up, allowing about 45cm (18in) turnover, *or* put on the duvet in its cover, overlapping the pillows and the foot of the bed.

4 Tuck in the sides of the top sheet and mitre the corners. Do the same with each blanket. Turn the top sheet down over the blankets and loosen the bed-clothes at the end of the bed to enable the patient to move his or her feet without restriction. Place the bedspread neatly on the bed.

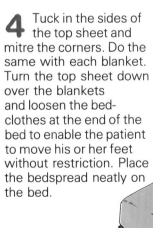
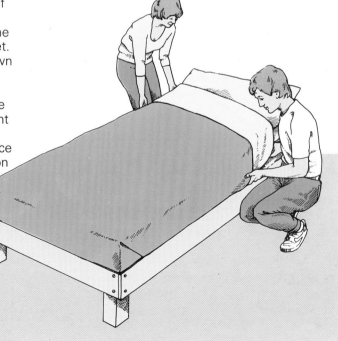

When a patient cannot get up

Explain how you are going to make the bed before you start or the patient may find the rolling distressing. Do not attempt this manoeuvre without help.

The room should be warm. Bring in any clean bed linen and put it on the chairs at the end of the bed. Have a laundry bag or bin ready.

Making the bed

1 Untuck the bed-clothes. Remove the upper layers and fold them neatly on to the chairs. Put them down in the order you will want them to remake the bed. Keep the patient covered with a blanket. Remove all but one pillow. Roll the clean sheet up length-wise and put it on top of the pile of bedclothes on the chairs. Roll the patient towards you. Support her while your helper rolls the soiled sheet up to the patient's back.

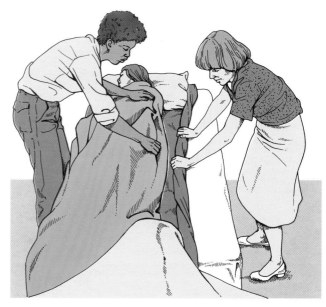

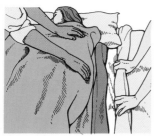

2 Support the patient on your side of the bed while your colleague straightens the under-blanket (and plastic sheet if one is being used) and tucks in the new sheet, unrolling it towards the patient's back.

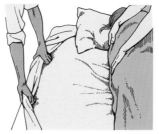

3 Your colleague rolls the patient over both sheets, supporting her while you remove the dirty sheet, straighten the underblanket and tuck in the new sheet. If you are using a fitted sheet, ease the corners into place.

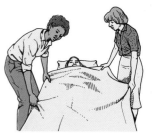

4 Take off the blanket. Replace the bed-clothes, with a clean top sheet or duvet cover if needed. Put on any clean pillowcases. Replace the pillows. Leave the patient in a comfortable position. Remove the dirty linen.

Drawsheets

Straightening the bed

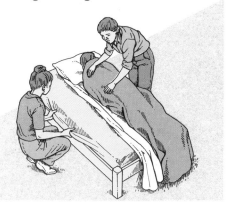

1 Follow the procedure described opposite up to removing the pillows. While your helper supports the patient on his side of the bed, untuck the bottom sheet and roll it up to the patient's back. Straighten the under-blanket, pull it taut and tuck it in.

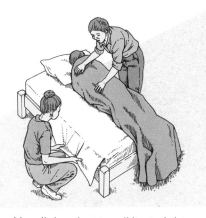

2 Unroll the sheet, pull it straight and tuck it in again.

3 Roll the patient towards you. Your helper should repeat the procedure on his side of the bed, Remove the blanket and replace the top bedclothes.

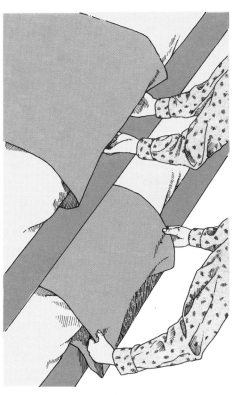

These can sometimes be useful for a patient who is feverish, perspiring and confined to bed. A drawsheet consists of a piece of material about 2m (6.5ft) long and 1m (3.3ft) wide — an old sheet folded in half lengthways is ideal. It goes on top of the sheet under the patient's bottom.

You adjust the drawsheet by un-tucking it both ends. Gently pull through a new part, giving the patient a fresh cool area of drawsheet without a major changing operation. This can be done several times because of its length. When it needs changing, do this the same way you change a sheet (see opposite). With incontinent patients, use incontinence pads not drawsheets.

Moving a patient

Take great care in lifting and moving a patient. If you lift the wrong way you may hurt yourself. Have someone to help you whenever possible. Remove anything on the floor you could trip over. Bend from the knees not the waist. Keep your back straight and wear low-heeled shoes or take them off. Lift towards you, never away and you will have better control. Remember to remove any jewellery which could scratch the patient's skin before you start. Always tell patients what you are going to do so that they can use their own muscle power as much as they can manage. Lift, don't drag, or you will damage the patient's skin and put pressure on a wound.

Moving a patient up a high bed

1 You and your helper face each other across the bed, knees slightly bent, one foot pointing at the bedhead. Clasp each other's near wrists (see far right) under the patients thighs.

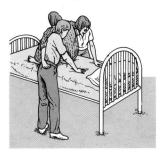
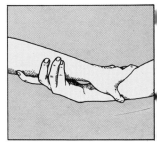

2 Put your other hands at the top of the mattress and lean inside shoulders against the patient's armpits.

3 Straighten your knees, pushing against the bed with your hands; put your weight on the feet nearest the bedhead, and move the patient up the bed as you do so. Keep up the pressure against the patient's armpits, so that she is held steady as you lift. It is best to lift on the count of three so that you work together. Get the patient to count too.

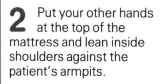
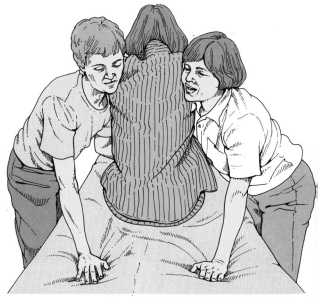

Moving a patient up a low bed

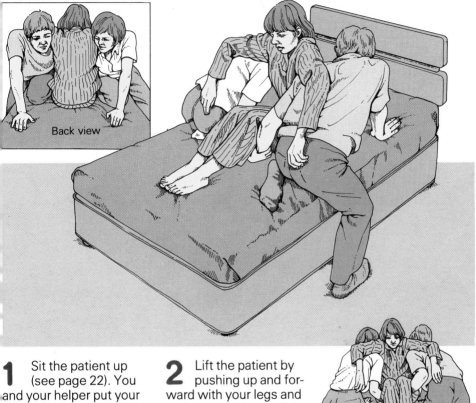

Back view

1 Sit the patient up (see page 22). You and your helper put your inner knees on the bed in line with the patient's hips. Grasp each other's wrists under the patient's thighs. Put your other hands further up the bed.

2 Lift the patient by pushing up and forward with your legs and taking part of her weight on your outer arms. Push against the patient's armpits with your shoulders and move up the bed in time with your helper.

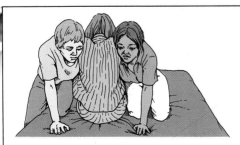

Moving up a double bed

Kneel on the bed, your knees by the patient's hips. Your helper has one foot on the floor, one on the bed. Working together, lift the patient up the bed as shown above. Press against her armpits, taking some weight on your outside arms.

Turning a patient in bed

A patient who is immobile to the extent of being unable to turn over should be turned by two people every couple of hours to prevent pressure sores. The lifting and turning must be done in one fluent movement to avoid strain on any of you. Remove the top bedclothes. The movements described here are for turning a patient to the right. Simply reverse them if you are turning a patient over to lie on his or her left side. Explain what you are going to do.

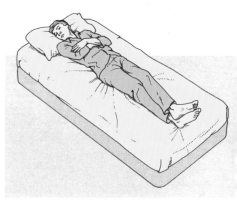

1 Turn the patient's head to the right. Cross his hands on to his chest and lift his left leg over the right.

2 Stand with your feet apart. Both put your hands under the patient's hips and shoulders. Grasp each other's wrists (see page 18).

3 Together gently ease the patient over the bed, lifting and turning him over on to the right side.

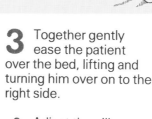

4 Adjust the pillows. Place the patient's arms in a comfortable position. Slightly bend the patient's legs and put a pillow under his upper leg.

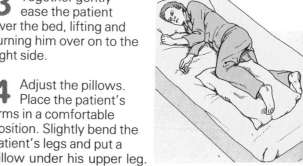

Moving a patient from bed to chair

Fairly immobile patients may still enjoy sitting in a chair for a while. A change of view, however slight, can be a morale boost. Unless a patient is critically ill, he or she should sit up out of bed for short periods each day, ideally for meals. The chair should be close to the bed so a minimum of lifting is needed. Talk the patient through the procedure before you start.

1 Raise him into a sitting position (see page 22). Ease his feet over the edge of the bed and help him into slippers and dressing gown.

2 You and your helper stand by the patient, one on either side. Grasp each other's nearer wrists under his thighs. Put your other hands and outer knees on the bed. Press your shoulders into his armpits (see left). With backs straight, bend at the knees and hips. With your shoulders firmly against the patient, press on the bed with your free hands, lifting as you straighten your knees.

3 Place your outside hands against the patient's back to support him. Move round slowly so you can turn away from the bed towards the chair (see above).

4 Grasp the chair arms with your outside hands and lower the patient into the chair.

Moving a patient alone

It cannot be too strongly emphasised that you can better assure the safety of the patient and yourself if you have help in moving him or her. However, there may be occasions when no-one else is available. You can still usually help a patient to get into a more comfortable position or to sit up.

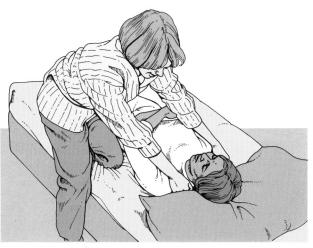

Sitting up

1 Put the patient's arms across her waist. Put your hands over her shoulders and your inner knee on the bed by her hip. Have your other foot on the floor in line with her waist.

2 Make sure your hands sufficiently cover her shoulders so that you will be able to support her when she is sitting up. Let your own weight raise the patient as you sit back on your heel keeping your arms straight. Arrange pillows or a backrest for her.

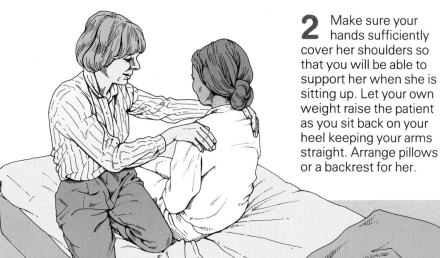

Turning a patient alone

If, unfortunately, you are left without help when an immobile patient needs turning, you must turn her on your own. If the patient is conscious, explain what you are going to do before you start.

Gently turn her head towards the left if you are turning to the left, remove the upper bedclothes and put her arms across her waist. Lift her right leg over her left leg. Place one hand under the patient's hips and the other under her shoulders, well forward. With straight back and knees bent, in one movement lift and turn the patient over. Arrange her arms and legs comfortably and put a pillow under her upper leg to cushion the bony parts. Replace the bedclothes and adjust the pillows.

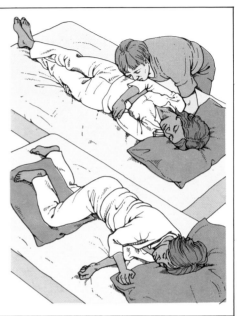

Moving up the bed

Sit the patient up. Get her to hold her wrist with her other hand and bend one leg. With your inner knee behind her buttocks and your weight on your other foot, hold her forearms from behind. Sit back. Your weight will carry her up the bed.

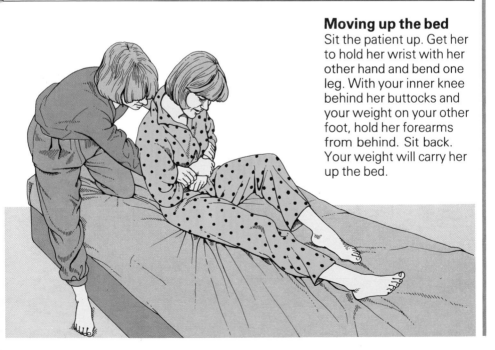

Comfort in bed

There are various different kinds of aids which are particularly helpful for patients who are confined to bed for a long time. The district nurse will advise about aids for special conditions.

Backrests can be very useful for patients who need support or who sit up for long periods. Some are shaped like the upper part of an armchair, others like a small upright deckchair. Triangular-shaped pillows can be helpful to sufferers from backache.

Orthopaedic bed boards placed under the mattress provide a firm support which helps patients with back problems who may be uncomfortable on soft beds. A large board or several smaller ones are equally effective.

Sheepskin pads help to relieve pressure and bed cradles (sometimes used with a blanket next to the skin) prevent bedclothes weighing on legs.

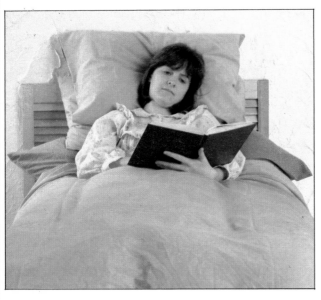

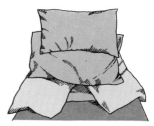

Pillows These can be banked up to support the patient in comfort. Put a pillow at the base of the bedhead, then stand two pillows leaning inward. Put another pillow across behind the small of the back and one on top to support head and shoulders.

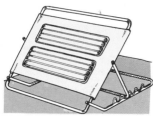

Backrests They are easy to use and with three pillows provide comfortable support.

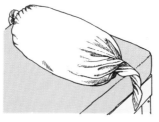

Footrests A pillow wrapped in a sheet supports the patient's feet at right angles.

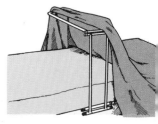

Bed cradles These help patients who have had a stroke, wound or burn on the lower body or legs.

Extra warmth

Try always to keep the patient's room at a comfortable temperature for him or her. If necessary try to supplement the heating with a thermostatically-controlled fan heater. But if extra warmth is needed in bed, try putting a cotton cellular blanket next to the patient's skin. Alternatively, use a rubber hot water bottle. Before filling it, make sure that it is in good condition and has a cover.

IMPORTANT

You should never allow patients to become severely chilled but it is dangerous to use hot water bottles for:
- **babies**
- **confused, very elderly or paralysed patients.**

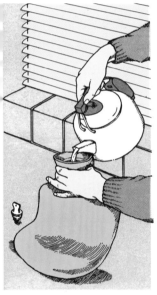

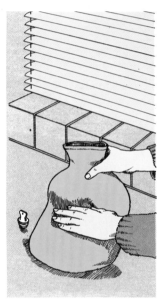

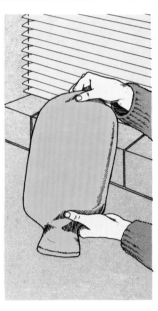

1 Put the hot water bottle flat on a surface and fill it two-thirds full of very hot, *not boiling* water. Do not pour too fast or the water may bubble up over your hand and scald you. Stand slightly to one side as you fill the hot water bottle so that the steam does not rise into your face.

2 Gently press out the air so that you can see the water at the neck of the bottle, before screwing in the stopper.

3 Turn the hot water bottle upside down to check it does not leak. Put it in a cover; a separate one is best as built-in covers leave the stopper exposed, which may burn. Put it over the first blanket if the patient has restricted movement or is elderly, or under a duvet wrapped in a towel.

Positions for bedrest

The patient's condition may indicate the best position for bedrest. For example: someone with breathing problems may only be comfortable well propped up, sitting or half sitting; someone with burns will not be able to tolerate any pressure on the affected part. Comfort and safety are the decisive factors, and a doctor or district nurse will advise you of any special requirements.

Half sitting

At least three pillows are used to prop up the patient (right). She can eat or read in comfort and may doze off knowing that she is well supported. She is upright enough to see around her.

Sitting up

A bank of pillows (above) or pillows and a backrest (see page 24), provide comfort for a patient sitting up. A foot support may be used if she is likely to slip down the bed and a bed cradle may help.

Lying flat

The patient may find that lying flat on her back is the most restful position. One or two pillows can support her head and unless her movement is restricted she can easily roll on to her side.

Pressure areas

When you are sitting or lying down, your weight presses down on the skin and tissue between your bones and the chair or bed. Healthy people are hardly aware of this at all because the nerve endings in the skin tell them to move automatically and frequently even in sleep. Patients who are unconscious or paralysed, very weak, elderly, thin or fat are most at risk of pressure sores (also known as bed sores) because movement may be impossible. The body weight may cut off the circulation to the tissue underneath. If neglected, the area becomes red, the tissue dies and breaks into an open wound: a pressure sore. The places these occur most commonly are the heels, the hips, the buttocks, elbows, shoulders and the back of the head, that is the bony parts most in contact with the bed.

Pressure areas

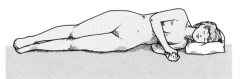

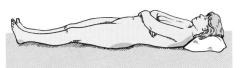

Prevention
It is much better to prevent a pressure sore than to try to cure it. Sores are less likely to develop if a patient eats a balanced diet and drinks enough (see pages 52–54). Encourage patients to move. Turn less mobile patients about every two hours. Gently massage vulnerable areas and exercise the joints

(the district nurse will tell you how). Keep the skin clean and dry. Remove any crumbs or bits from the bed, pulling the bottom sheet taut. Always lift the patient carefully, avoiding any friction on the skin.

Particular care should be taken with patients who are paralysed or incontinent. Barrier cream may be used to help protect the skin. Natural or artificial sheepskin can be placed under the buttocks or shoulders to relieve pressure. Well-placed pillows are useful too but take advice from the district nursing sister/charge nurse, for if they are used wrongly problems are created.

Treatment
Pressure sores are wounds which may be extremely painful and very difficult to heal. There are various ointments available on prescription and more sophisticated methods of treatment for which expert advice is required. A doctor or district nurse should be consulted about pressure sores. It is essential to turn regularly, to maintain high standards of hygiene and to improve the patient's condition.

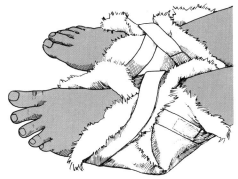

Sheepskin protection
Bootees ease pressure on the patient's heels.

Personal care

Helping to keep a patient clean is a very important part of your nursing care. Perspiration drying on the skin may make it sore and smell unpleasant. A bath or all-over wash once a day will refresh the patient and give you an ideal opportunity to check on his or her condition, to change a dressing on a wound or attend to other skin care. Any adverse changes in the skin must be reported to the district nurse or doctor.

It is essential to maintain the highest standards of cleanliness with someone who is ill. If the surroundings are not hygienic, the patient's body must fight infection from dirt as well as sickness or injury.

Your care may include shaving a patient and helping to look after hair, nails, mouth and eyes. How much help is needed will vary with the individual. Find out how much help a patient requires when dressing or undressing or with any part of a wash, and how often he or she usually baths.

A feverish patient (one with a raised temperature) will perspire more heavily, becoming hot, sticky and

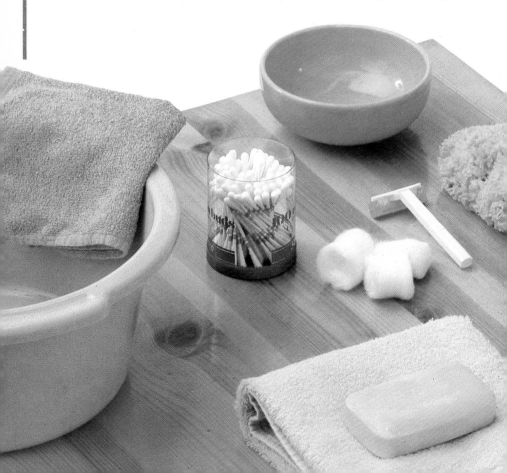

uncomfortable. Regular sponging down or bathing is essential for cleanliness and plays an important part in bringing his or her temperature down.

Face and hands
Besides a daily bath or all-over wash, a patient may find that washing the face and hands several times a day is very refreshing, particularly if he or she has a raised temperature. The patient will also need to wash his or her hands after using a commode or bedpan and before meals. If a patient cannot get out of bed, offer a bowl of warm water, soap, a flannel and towel.

Encourage the person you are looking after to attend to his or her general appearance if possible. If not, you must do it as such care is a boost to the patient's morale and to that of the rest of the family.

The bathroom

If the patient can use the bathroom, make it as safe and pleasant as possible. See that the windows are closed and that the room is warm enough. Place within easy reach the toiletries and clean clothes the patient may need. Run the cold water into the bath first, then add the hot, until the water temperature is comfortable.

You may be needed to help the patient along to the bathroom, undress, go to the lavatory, get in or out of the bath and dress afterwards.

Less mobile patients should use a bath seat (see page 85). It is unwise for the patient to lock the door and you should stay within call. Never leave a young child or someone who has had a stroke alone in the bath.

Showers
A shower is usually quicker than a bath and may be easier to get in and out of for someone with limited mobility. It is worth investing in thermostatic control or an anti-scald safeguard. A shower seat will prevent the patient from becoming exhausted (see p. 85).

Giving a bed bath

Patients who cannot get up will need to have an all-over wash in bed once a day. See that the bedroom is warm. Tell the patient what you are going to do and place the equipment you will need by the bed. Ask if the patient wishes to use a bedpan first. Remove the top bedclothes and the patient's clothing. Place a towel under each part as you wash it to protect the bed and keep the patient covered as much as possible with the other towel. Check that the water is warm. Change it as it cools and after washing around the genital area.

You will need:
- bowl of warm water
- two large towels
- soap
- two flannels
- toiletries
- clean clothing
- brush and comb
- toothbrush, tooth-
paste, mug, denture pot
- razor.

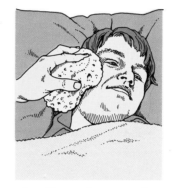

1 The patient may like to wash, rinse and dry his own hands, face and neck if he is able. If not, do it for him.

2 Wash, rinse and dry each arm, from arm-pit to wrist, then his ches and abdomen (tummy). Use a deodorant or talcum powder under the arms if the patient wishes

3 Wash, rinse and dry the legs and feet. Many patients prefer to wash the groin and geni-tal area themselves if they can manage. If not, you must do it. This can be done without exposing the area and is easier if the patient lies on one side. Change the water.

4 Wash the patient's back with him lying on his side facing you so that you can provide sup-port (see left).

5 Help the patient into clean clothes (see pages 34–35). Provide cold water for cleaning his teeth and hot water for shaving and help if needed. Remake the bed, make the patient comfortable and offer to brush and comb his hair.

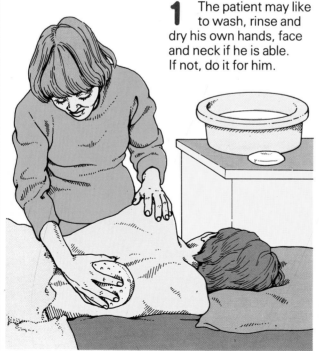

Hair care

The patient's hair should be brushed and combed several times a day at least. When a patient can cope, provide a brush, comb and mirror. If you comb hair for the patient, ask where to put a parting. Patients who are ill for long will need their hair washing. If they are mobile enough to use the bathroom, hair can be washed in the usual way. A local hairdresser may be prepared to come in when necessary and such a visit might prove a boost to morale.

However, hair can be attended to without difficulty even when the patient is in bed by dry shampooing or damp washing. Remember to protect the patient's shoulders and the bed with towels and to use a clean brush and comb afterwards. Wash the patient's brush and comb in a weak solution of antiseptic. Rinse and dry them thoroughly before use.

Dry shampooing
This causes minimal disturbance to the patient. Cover the hair with the shampoo powder and be sure to brush it out thoroughly, following the instructions on the container.

Damp washing
This can be done whatever position the patient is nursed in. Protect the bedding by slipping a towel under the patient's head and shoulders. Put a bowl of warm water nearby on a protected surface. Dampen a sponge or flannel and use it to massage the scalp well and rub the hair. Do this to the whole head. Check with the patient that you are not pressing too hard. Use a hair dryer if possible or rub the hair gently with a warm towel. When the hair is quite dry, brush and comb it so that it feels comfortable and looks neat.

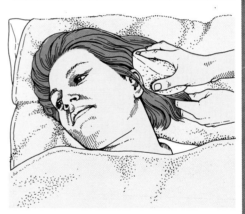

Caring for nails

The patient's toenails and fingernails must be kept clean and may need cutting. Cut fingernails or file and round them to the shape of the finger. Cut toenails straight across. Elderly patients sometimes suffer from hard and uncomfortable toenails and may be helped by a chiropodist who can be contacted through the local health authority or social services.

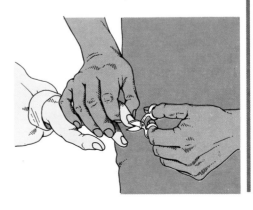

Care of the mouth

When we eat tiny bits of food remain in the mouth afterwards. These particles start to decompose, bacteria flourish and can cause tooth decay unless teeth are cleaned regularly.

A high fluid intake helps to keep the mouth fresh. Leave a water jug within the patient's reach. The sharp flavour of fresh fruit juices is very refreshing and so are mild antiseptic mouthwashes. They encourage the production of saliva (fluid in the mouth) which helps to keep the mouth clean and fresh.

Many patients who cannot get up may be able to brush their own teeth in bed. If they can, offer a toothbrush (a battery-operated one is ideal) and tooth paste, a glass of water, a bowl to spit into and a towel in the morning and last thing in the evening. If the patient cannot clean his or her own mouth, you must do it, before and after meals. Tuck a towel under the patient's chin, explaining what you will be doing.

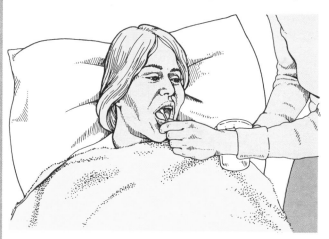

Cleaning the mouth

Dip cotton wool buds into a container of bicarbonate of soda solution (5ml to a tumbler of warm water). Gently clean all the surfaces of the mouth. Use fresh cotton wool buds dipped in mouthwash to remove the taste of the solution. Offer water for the patient to rinse out her mouth and a bowl to spit into or flavoured buds which freshen the mouth

Cleaning dentures

These should be cleaned at least twice a day. Ask the patient to put them in a container. Brush them well under running water using a denture cleanser. Special denture cream or powder can be used if they are stained. Before giving them back to the patient, rinse them thoroughly. Dentures can be left in water or cleaning solution overnight.

Children's teeth

Make sure that children know that cleaning teeth after meals is important. Get them into the habit as soon as possible, perhaps by making teeth-cleaning into a game.

When a child has a few teeth, buy a soft toothbrush. Show him or her how to move it over the surface of the teeth to remove bits of food left after meals.

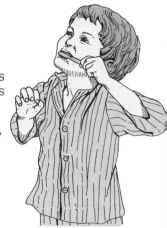

Bathing a baby

Make sure the room is warm. To wash the baby use water which feels warm to your elbow, about 30°C (85°F). When the baby is very young moisten cotton wool balls and gently swab the face and hands. Use a new swab for each part and clean the nappy area with cotton wool and baby lotion. This "topping and tailing" cleans the important bits and means that the young baby needs a full bath only every other day. Talk to and play with the baby.

You will need within reach:
- baby soap, baby shampoo, baby lotion
- cotton wool swabs
- bag for used swabs
- clean clothing, clean nappy
- soft flannel or sponge
- large towel
- laundry bag or bucket.

Fill the baby bath with cold water first then hot to reach the correct warmth.

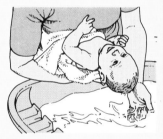

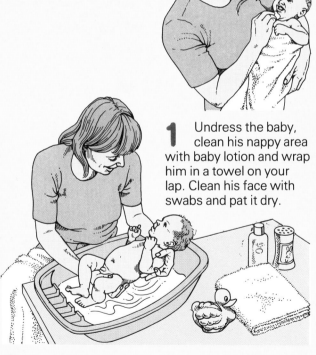

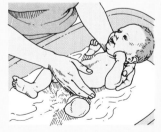

1 Undress the baby, clean his nappy area with baby lotion and wrap him in a towel on your lap. Clean his face with swabs and pat it dry.

2 Hold the baby along your arm. Cradle his head on one hand and wash his hair. Rinse and pat dry. Use shampoo only about once a week.

3 Support his head and shoulders on one hand and forearm, with his bottom and the thigh furthest from you on your other hand as you lower him into the water. Keep his head and neck well supported. Smile and talk to him, making bath time fun so that he enjoys the water.

4 Use your free hand to wash and rinse him. Lift him out carefully. Wrap him in the towel and pat him dry. Check his skin creases are dry.

Clothes

Choice of clothing is such a personal matter that any help you give a patient in choosing what to wear or in dressing or undressing should be offered as tactfully as possible. Always make sure patients are warmly dressed because someone who is inactive feels the cold more than those who can move around and take exercise.

Dressing is a slower process for someone with limited movement or sight, so keep the room warm. While you should be available if help is needed, encourage patients to do as much as possible themselves to boost their independence and morale.

There are many ways in which clothing can be simplified if the patient's condition is long-lasting. Back fastenings and tight-fitting garments should be avoided if the patient has only limited movement. Pockets at the front are much more accessible than ones at the side for someone who is sitting down most of the time. Front-fastening bras and wrap-over skirts can be a boon to a

Dressing and undressing

Patients may be embarrassed by your presence. Be assuring, talk through the procedures and let patients help themselves, however slow and minimal their efforts might be.

Work at a pace the patient can cope with, resting when necessary. If the patient is unsteady, make sure he or she is comfortably supported before putting anything over the head, putting on or removing tights, stockings or footwear. Do up buttons and zips as you go but leave waistband fastenings until last so that you can tuck in a shirt easily. The top part of the body should be dressed first and undressed last. Be gentle in your movements and pull the clothes not the patient.

Helping with trousers
Slip the trousers over the patient's feet (below) and ease them up. Help him raise his bottom. Pull the trousers up (right). Do up the zip.

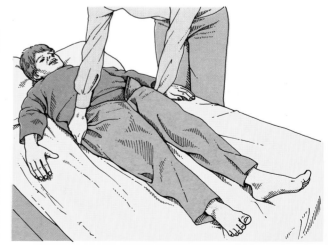

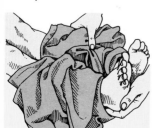

woman with arthritic hands or re-cuperating after a stroke. Lace-up shoes give good support and elastic laces may enable patients to put them on without help. Simple dressing aids are very useful (see page 84). Velcro strips can be inserted in trouser seams if zips cause difficulty and ties can be permanently knotted if they are cut at the back and Velcro fasteners put in. Clothing should be made of easy-care fabric which is simple to wash and needs little or no ironing.

Clothes to wear in bed

These should be comfortable and loose-fitting. Cotton is the ideal material because it absorbs perspiration well. Many of the cotton and synthetic mixtures are also acceptable and are very easy to wash. Patients should wear the kind of nightdress or pyjamas they find most comfortable. Men might find nightshirts easier than pyjamas to get in and out of while they are ill. Track suits are a happy compromise between nightclothes and getting fully dressed.

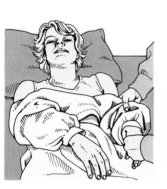
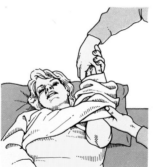

Helping with a nightdress *Either* ease her arms into the sleeves (far left) and then gently put the neck opening over her head, easing the garment down; *or* put the nightdress over her head, then over her arms (left).

Helping with sleeves Always deal with an injured or paralysed arm first. Reach through and grasp the patient's hand and draw the sleeve up her arm.

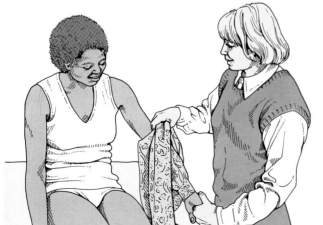
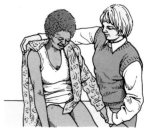

Baby clothes

Although they are fairly immobile, small babies are far from clean. They dribble and bring up milk and there will be leaks from nappies. So they need frequent changing. They grow very rapidly in the first months and clothing will be quickly outgrown but the parents should buy enough easy-care washable garments. Clothing should keep the baby comfortably warm without restricting movement. Keep it simple. The fewer ribbons and strings to tie the better; both you and the baby will find dressing and undressing quicker and less upsetting without them. All-in-one stretch suits are particularly convenient but remember that not even stretch material grows with the baby.

Select clothing that opens down the front or has a wide neckline because babies hate to have things pulled over their faces. Raglan sleeves will allow you to put your hand in to guide the baby's arm through. All clothes should allow easy access to the nappy so that a minimum of undressing is necessary. Stretch suits should have poppers at the crutch or all down the front and legs. Avoid garments with lacy holes which catch the baby's fingers and avoid too much white; once a child is crawling it will quickly look grubby and

Dressing a baby

Many newborn babies feel insecure being naked, disliking the air on their skin. You may feel worried, too, by the difficulty of handling this vulnerable creature, supporting a wobbly head and getting the baby in or out of clothing. Practice and gentleness will result in growing confidence so that it can be accomplished with very little fuss. Stay calm. If the baby is very distressed, do not leave him or her uncovered; try putting a clean nappy over the tummy – the contact may have a soothing effect. Dress a new baby on a flat surface.

Dressing

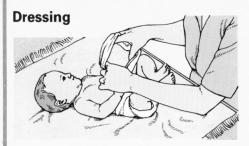

1 Settle the baby on a changing mat or soft rug on the flat surface. This leaves your hands free. Stretch the neck of the vest and carefully put it over her head.

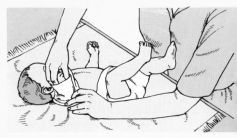

2 Put your hand up the sleeve to stretch it and guide her arm through, repeat with her other arm. Pull down the vest. Repeat with other garments that go over the baby's head.

brighter colours are more stimulating.

If a baby is kicking strongly, a baby sleeping bag is a practical way of ensuring that he or she stays warm and covered. Always cover a baby's head with a hat outside in cold weather. Toddlers need warm outdoor clothing such as mini track suits or dungarees.

How many of anything the parents buy is up to them and to the time of year. If the baby is born in the summer, they will not need to buy mittens for outdoors but will need a sun hat. Other clothes will probably be cotton. A winter baby might need wool cardigans, a thicker shawl and a wool hat.

The baby will need:
- all-in-one stretch suits
- wide-necked vests
- cardigans or jumpers
- nightdresses
- mittens
- socks
- hats
- shawl for swaddling
- sleeping bag
- warm outdoor gear.

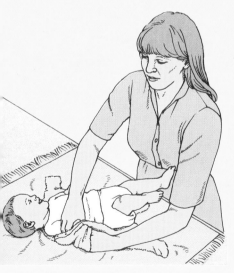

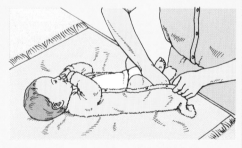

4 Ease the baby's right leg down so that her foot goes down to the end of the suit and repeat with the other leg. Do up all the poppers.

Undressing
Simply reverse the process. First lay the baby on the flat surface, then ease her out of her clothes. Always be careful to pull the clothing rather than the baby. Immediately wrap her in a towel and cuddle her so that she feels warm and secure.

3 If you are using a stretch suit, open it out flat and lay the baby on top. Gather up the sleeve, reach through for her hand and pull the sleeve up her arm. Repeat with the other arm.

Elimination

Your practical knowledge and tactful care are extremely important in helping patients to deal with their excretions (elimination). They may be very embarrassed and find it hard to accept your help. Never show embarrassment, impatience or reluctance, for your priority is always to protect patients' dignity, to respect their privacy and to be sensitive in your handling, even when a patient is unconscious. When patients are not very mobile or do not have full control of their bladder or bowel, for example, after a stroke, they may be very anxious and upset. Your calm practical approach can do much to allay such fears.

A woman of child-bearing age may need your tactful assistance in coping with her monthly period. Supply tampons or sanitary towels as needed and dispose of soiled ones.

Saving a specimen
Occasionally a district nurse or doctor might ask you to take a specimen and you would be told how to do this. Such an excretion might be of urine (water), faeces (solid waste), vomit (sick) or sputum (fluid coughed up from the lungs). You will be provided with a suitable container. You should write clearly on the label giving the patient's name, address, the nature of the contents, the date and time.

General hygiene
Empty bedpans, urinals or commode containers down the toilet. Using a cloth kept only for that purpose rinse them out with cold water and a mild antiseptic. Always wash your hands after helping with the patient's excretions. Remove vomit, urine or faeces from the bedroom as soon as possible and disperse unpleasant smells by opening a window and using an air-freshening spray.

Sputum
A healthy person's sputum is usually clear and frothy. Infected sputum is thick and yellow/green. If a patient is coughing up a lot of sputum, provide a good supply of tissues by the bed and a waxed carton or plastic container with a lid such as a yoghurt pot. Encourage the patient to spit into the carton or cough into a tissue. Provide a bin for the tissues. Sputum contains organisms which may be a source of infection so keep containers covered. Clear away paper handkerchiefs and containers regularly. Wrap them in newspaper or put them into a polythene bag and seal it, then put them in the dustbin or burn them. The doctor may suggest inhalations (see page 51).

IMPORTANT

Observe the patient's excretions carefully. Seek medical help if:
- **vomiting is accompanied by diarrhoea**
- **you are worried about the frequency, colour or concentration of urine**
- **you are concerned about a bottle-fed baby's stools — the formula may need changing.**

Pause to think whether colour changes could be due to diet: for example, eating spinach or drinking blackcurrant cordial may make faeces dark or urine red.

Vomiting

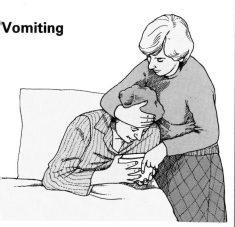

A patient who has vomited or who just feels sick is often distressed and very uncomfortable. Children may be frightened and you can do much to comfort them. Encourage deep breathing.

Get a bowl and some kitchen paper immediately a patient feels sick. If the patient starts to retch, remove any false teeth if possible. Hold the bowl steady or let the patient do this while you support his or her head. Cover the bedclothes with the kitchen paper if you can and use it to clear away any soiling. Remove the vomit from the bedroom at once and flush it down the lavatory. Help the patient to wash his or her face and hands. Provide a mouthwash, and water to drink if the patient wants it. Change the patient's bedding and clothes if necessary.

If the vomit is other than water or undigested food, put a specimen in a clean covered container somewhere cool and retain it for the doctor. Note the patient's pulse rate and colour, the time of sickness, whether it was linked with eating, drinking or medicines and whether the patient felt pain.

Make sure the patient is warm and put the washed bowl back by the bed.

Faeces

We absorb the nutrients from the food we eat while it is in the stomach and intestines. Any remaining undigested matter is expelled from the bowel, in adults usually as semi-solid brown stools. If a patient's stools are different from the normal appearance, tell the doctor or district nurse who may ask you to save a specimen. Adults usually pass faeces about once a day but individual habits vary a great deal.

A newborn baby passes a greeny stool which changes, becoming light brown, then probably bright yellow by around the third week. Breast-fed babies normally continue to pass loose yellowish stools while bottle-fed babies usually produce a more formed stool. The stools become more adult as the baby is weaned.

Diarrhoea

A patient who passes soft watery stools at frequent intervals has diarrhoea. He or she may become very ill from dehydration (fluid loss) if severe diarrhoea continues and a baby can die in hours. Tell the doctor about the condition right away. Save a specimen if this is possible.

Constipation

This occurs when the usual pattern is disrupted for some reason and the bowel does not empty. Healthy people sometimes get constipation from eating too little fibre or not drinking enough fluids. Adjusting the diet often cures the problem (see page 53). Constipation is a common problem among people who are ill. If the condition lasts for a week or if it causes real discomfort, consult the patient's doctor or the district nurse.

Daily excretions

Find out how able patients are to cope with their own excretions, how much help will be needed from you and roughly at what times you will be wanted. Most people have some routine and like to keep to this. It is usual to pass urine soon after waking, before meals and before going to sleep at night.

If the patient can get to a lavatory you may just be wanted to provide a supporting hand. Remain within call. If he or she can get out of bed but not out of the room, a commode will be needed; bedbound patients will require a bedpan and urinal.

Using a commode
Close the bedroom door and help the patient to sit up and put on slippers and dressing gown. Remove the cover of the commode, move it close to the bed and help the patient to get pyjamas or nightdress out of the way. When the patient is sitting on the commode it is a good idea to put a blanket over his or her lap to provide extra warmth and reduce embarrassment. Place a roll of

toilet paper within easy reach and unless the patient is weak or confused, leave the room but remain within call. The patient should wash his or her hands afterwards. If there is no basin in the room, provide a bowl of warm water, soap and a towel before helping the patient back to bed. A bedpan placed on a chair is an acceptable alternative if there is no commode.

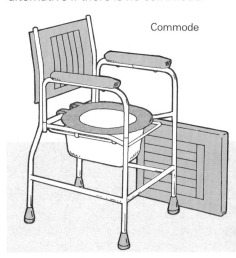

Commode

Incontinence

This is the term used for the inability to control the passing of urine or faeces. It can happen at any age after injury, or may be due to infection, stress or to degeneration in old age. The involuntary loss of control over the muscles of the bladder or bowel may be acutely upsetting and embarrassing for the patient. The district nurse or doctor can advise about special incontinence aids and about the financial and practical help available from the social services.

Urinary incontinence
This is common to all of us as babies when the bladder empties at once and involuntarily. By early childhood we have usually learnt control but it is sometimes temporarily lost due to an emotional or physical shock. Incontinence is commonest among elderly people. Regular visits to the toilet and garments that are easy to remove in a hurry will help. Stress incontinence is sometimes a problem for women

Urinals

These are differently shaped for men and women. They are very useful for seriously ill patients and can be used with very little disturbance. Take the urinal to the bed covered with a piece of kitchen roll or paper towel. Give it to the patient or put it in place. Provide lavatory paper, cleaning the patient if he or she cannot use it. Cover the urinal and take it from the room. If there is no urinal, a wide-topped jar can be used for men and a bedpan for women. Again, the patient's hands and your own will need washing. Wash out the urinal or other container.

Giving a bedpan

Close the bedroom door and see that the bedpan is warm and dry. Cover it with a piece of kitchen paper or paper towel. Take it and a roll of lavatory paper to the bedside. Help to move pyjamas or nightdress out of the way and to raise the patient so that you can slide the bedpan under the buttocks. You may need a helper. If the patient is able to sit up, using a bedpan is much easier. Afterwards offer the lavatory paper, or if the patient cannot use it you should attend to this. Remove the bedpan and cover it. Straighten the bedclothes and provide the patient with the means to wash his or her hands. Leave the patient in a comfortable position and take the bedpan from the room to clean it.

Bedpan

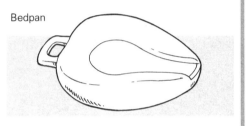

Male urinal

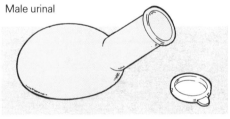

before and after childbirth when the womb may press on the bladder. Older men sometimes become incontinent due to an enlarged prostate gland. Both these conditions can usually be cured by an operation if they become severe. Stroke patients sometimes become incontinent but may regain control.

Damage to the spinal cord may deprive someone of bladder and bowel control permanently. Faecal incontinence is rare in other cases.

Treatment

The patient should drink sufficiently – restricting the liquid intake (except at night) may make incontinence worse not better. The diet should contain roughage (fibre), vegetables and fruit so that the patient is not constipated. When leakages occur, gently wash and dry the skin and put on a barrier cream. Remove soiled bedclothes and bedding. Be prompt, unembarrassed and sensitive in your attentions.

Nappies

There are many diffferent kinds of nappies and ways of putting them on. Use only special nappy safety pins to fasten nappies, keep your hand between safety pins and the baby's skin when changing and never put down an open pin.

Types of nappy

You will need to decide whether to use washable nappies or disposables or perhaps a combination.

The basic washable nappy is a terry towelling square which is quick drying and very absorbent when folded to give several thicknesses where there is most wetness. Muslin nappy liners are very soft and can be used on their own for the newborn's first week. Specially shaped towelling nappies are soft and need no folding but are expensive and take longer to dry.

Disposable nappies are absorbent pads that are plastic-backed or worn in plastic holders. They are not as absorbent as terry nappies but you avoid laundry problems. Disposables can be bought in different sizes.

One-way liners are used next to the skin, with a nappy. They are made of material that lets through urine one way but not back, so the baby stays drier.

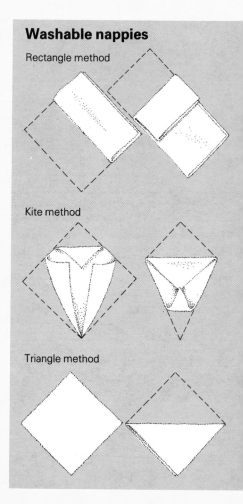

Washable nappies

Rectangle method

Kite method

Triangle method

Changing nappies

Never leave a baby in a wet or soiled nappy. Whenever a nappy needs changing, put the baby down on a soft mat on a flat surface. Have everything you want within reach. Remove the old nappy, using it to wipe away any soiling. Clean the buttocks with mild soap and water or cotton wool and baby lotion or baby oil. Dry the area gently and apply a soothing barrier cream to prevent nappy rash. Lift the baby's bottom by raising his or her ankles in one hand, keeping one finger between to stop them rubbing. Fold a terry nappy in one of the ways shown above. Slip the new nappy under the baby, bringing the top up to waist level. Fasten a disposable with its tabs and a terry nappy as shown opposite. Always wash your hands after you have been handling dirty nappies.

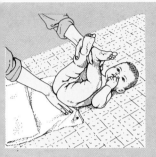 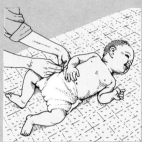

Rectangle method
This is good with small babies. Fold the nappy in half (see far left). Fold up the bottom third for a boy, fold down the top for a girl. Lay the baby on it. Bring up the lower part. Pin at the hips.

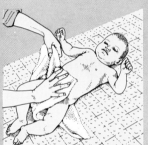 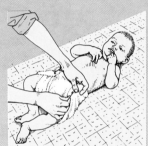

Kite method
This is good for all sizes of baby. Fold in the two side corners, bring the top flap over and the bottom point up (see far left). Put the baby on the nappy. Bring up the part between the legs and pin at each hip.

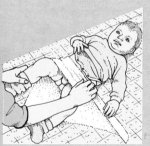 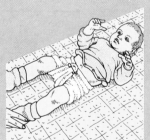

Triangle method
This is good with big babies. Fold the nappy in half to form a triangle. Fold down the top edge (see far left). Put the baby on the nappy. Bring the sides over. Bring up the point, pin in the middle.

Disposable nappies

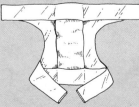

Tie-on with separate pad

Popper pants with separate pad

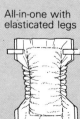

All-in-one with elasticated legs

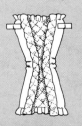

All-in-one with shaped legs

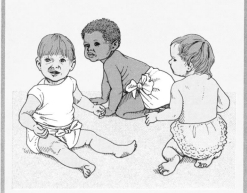

Sterilising nappies

Nappies must be sterilised to remove all traces of urine and faeces in order to avoid infection and skin irritation, then rinsed very well.

Special nappy sterilants considerably reduce the chore of washing nappies, which otherwise need to be boiled. There should be two big plastic buckets with lids, different colours so you can tell them apart. Fill both with fresh nappy-sterilising solution every morning. Put wet nappies in one, soiled nappies in the other, first shaking the worst of the solid matter into the lavatory. Add wet and soiled nappies to the respective buckets throughout the day. Nappies are sterilised only after they have been submerged for six hours. Put nappies you change in the night in a plastic bag, ready to be soaked the next day.

The sterilising solution must be changed every 24 hours. When you discard the old mixture in the morning, the "wet" nappies do not need washing with detergent. Just rinse them thoroughly. The ones that were soiled should be washed in very hot water with pure soap flakes, mild detergent or low lather powder, then thoroughly rinsed or the baby may get nappy rash.

Dry nappies outside if you can or in a tumble drier. Do not put them on hot pipes or radiators because they will then feel stiff and hard against a baby's soft skin.

Nappy sterilants are poisonous — keep them away from children. They also contain bleach, so never put a coloured garment in even if it is soiled. Wash solution off your hands before touching the baby's sensitive skin and if you find that it irritates your own skin, wear rubber gloves.

Plastic pants

These are necessary with most disposable nappies and may be used with terry nappies. There are various designs. Wetness is retained so check that you are not keeping clothes and bedding dry at the cost of a red sore bottom. Plastic pants which tie at the side are a good compromise in that they provide protection but do allow a little evaporation and air circulation. If they become wet or soiled, wash them in warm water with a mild detergent. Rinse and dry them well.

Nappy rash

Sometimes a baby gets sore reddened buttocks, usually from remaining in a wet nappy or because nappies have been inadequately rinsed. Leave off plastic pants and if possible let the baby lie on an unfastened nappy for a while. Change wet nappies as soon as possible and apply zinc and castor oil cream to soothe the skin and form a waterproof barrier. Consult your doctor if the condition persists. Be extra thorough about how you wash and rinse the baby's nappies. A baby with a sore nappy rash will probably cry more than usual. Be specially gentle and soothing with him or her.

Control of bowel and bladder

Managing bowel and bladder movements by conscious control is a skill a child learns gradually. Movements are automatic until the age of about 15 months. Some time in the second year of life a child recognises the connection between the sensation of passing urine and faeces and the result. Control can now be learned.

Bowel movements

These are easier to predict and control than the bladder so the child will probably learn to use the potty for them first. He or she may make obvious signs that a motion is imminent, perhaps suddenly standing still, clutching at a nappy and making a sound in anticipation. If you are watching for such signs, you can suggest that the child might like to sit on the potty so that the faeces go in there. Be gentle and low key in your approach. Do not insist that the pot is used but be quietly pleased when it is and the desired result is achieved.

Bladder control

This is more difficult and takes longer because a child urinates so many times a day and the interval between knowing that a motion is coming and the flood being produced is very short. If the child is dry after an afternoon nap, suggest sitting on the potty to have a pee. Congratulate successes. Start leaving off nappies and buy some plastic-backed terry towelling trainer pants which are easy to take down in a hurry. A sudden clenching of the buttocks or standing rigid with crossed legs are the usual signs of urgent need for the pot. There will be frequent puddles and accidents in the beginning. You should treat these with sympathy and mop up with minimal fuss or the pot will be associated with tension and failure. The child may still need nappies at night for a year or so and many children are occasionally wet at night until they are five. If a child continues to be wet after that age, a doctor or health visitor may be able to help.

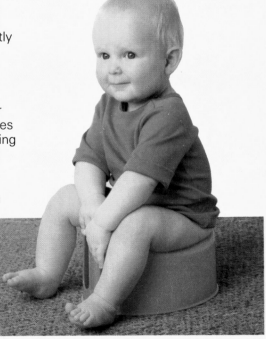

Using a potty
Buy a potty which is easy to clean and unlikely to tip up when the child wriggles. He should feel comfy and secure on it. Never scold a child for not getting to the pot in time.

Daily routines

What happens and when in daily care depends very much on how ill the patient is, the nature of the illness, the patient's own wishes and when help is available. Some routine is important so that medicines, meals and any special care are given at the right time and according to the patient's medical and nursing instructions.

Observing the patient

Sometimes you might be asked to take a patient's pulse or temperature, or check the rate of breathing. Remember that the patient should be sitting or lying quietly for any of these observations. You should use an accurate watch or clock with a second hand to count by. You may be given special charts on which to keep records. Keep such records of the patient's progress together to give to the doctor or district nurse when they call.

You will probably be spending more time with the patient than the other people involved in his or her medical care. You will have opportunities to watch the patient and see if he or she is

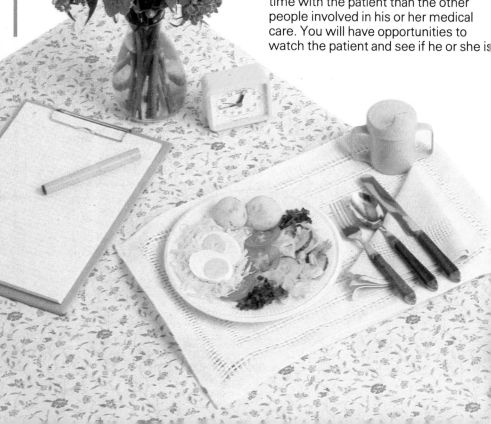

1 pain, worried or not eating and if
here is any change in condition. Your
observations enable you to respond
promptly to the patient's needs.

Occupying the patient

Remember that a prolonged stay in bed
is very boring. If the patient is well
enough to appreciate the radio, books,
telephone, newspapers, or other
entertainment, try to provide these. A
remote control television can be a
wonderful aid in passing the time.

Your company may mean much to
the patient. You can offer reassurance
to someone who is anxious, and do
make time to play with a sick child or
read to him or her. Relax the rules if the
condition allows, giving his or her
favourite foods and perhaps a couple
of new toys. Ill children particularly
need love and attention to comfort
them while they feel unwell. Explain in
simple terms what the illness is so that
a child can understand.

People tire more easily when they
are sick, and periods of rest are just as
essential as stimulation. Visitors may
be very welcome but they should not
stay for too long.

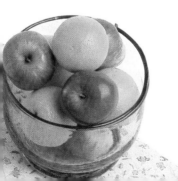

Taking a temperature

Normal body temperature is usually
considered to be in the range 36–37°C
(97–99°F). Injury or infection may cause
it to rise. Hypothermia is the term given
to a dangerous fall below normal.
Taking the temperature is a useful
guide to the patient's condition.

The mouth is usually the most reli-
able and convenient place to take a
temperature; if it is taken in the armpit
it will be slightly lower, so you should
make a note of the method used. You
may want to practise taking a temperature to be confident of reading the
mercury in a clinical thermometer. The
thermometer should be kept in its case,
or in an empty glass. Disposable or re-
usable thermometers are less accurate
but they are easy to use, safe and
particularly convenient with babies,
children, elderly or confused patients.
You should not take the temperature by
mouth in some cases (see page 49).

Thermometers

A clinical mercury-filled thermometer is the most accurate sort.
Many show both fahrenheit and
centigrade. Re-usable strip thermometers are put on the forehead
and show the temperature in
30 seconds. Disposable thermometers (not shown) and re-usable
strips are safest with children.

Clinical mercury-filled thermometer

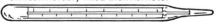

Re-usable strip thermometer

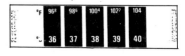

°F	96⁸	98⁶	100⁴	102²	104
°C	36	37	38	39	40

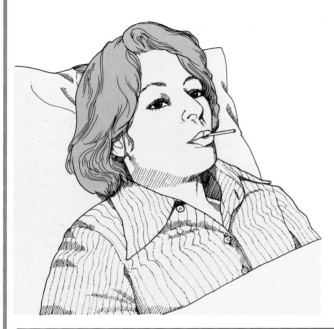

By mouth

1 Rinse the thermo-
meter under the col*
tap, dry it and check that
the mercury is shaken
down into the bulb.

2 Put the thermo-
meter in the
patient's mouth under he*
tongue. Ask her to close
her lips but not her teeth.

3 After one minute
remove the thermo-
meter, wipe it, read and
record the temperature.
Shake down the mercury*
Put the thermometer
away safely.

Pulse

With each heartbeat we can feel a
pulse throb wherever a large artery is
near the surface, for example, the
wrist. Adults usually have a pulse rate
of 60 to 80 beats per minute when at
rest. Heart disease, shock, infection,
exercise, tension and emotion are
among the possible causes of a high
pulse rate. Hypothermia or certain

drugs might cause the pulse to beat
more slowly than usual.
   The thumb and fingertips have
pulses so use the pads of your fingers
to take a pulse to avoid confusion.
Practise taking your own pulse or that
of a friend. Remember to note the rate,
strength and rhythm. A normal pulse is
quite strong and has a regular rhythm.

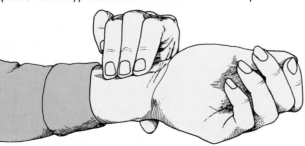

Taking a pulse
To check the pulse rate at
the wrist, feel the inside of
the wrist on the thumb side,
just up from the creases
between hand and forearm.
Hold the patient's wrist with
your fingerpads on the
pulse; count the beats for
one minute. Write the
number down.

Giving medicines

If you are looking after someone at home, you may be asked to give the patient medicines by mouth or by inhalation (breathed in). Medicines are given as injections by a nurse or doctor except in the case of patients with diabetes who may inject themselves with insulin. Even simple cold remedies can cause side-effects such as drowsiness, so handle all medicines with the greatest care — they may be dangerous if they are misused. Follow exactly any instructions given by the doctor. If you ever have charge of a prescription, check that the chemist gives you the right person's medicine. There are four rules you must follow. Give:

- the right amount
- of the right medicine
- at the right time
- to the right patient.

IMPORTANT

Do not take the temperature in the mouth when:

- **the patient cannot breathe through his or her nose or has breathing problems**
- **the patient is a young child**
- **the patient has a mouth injury or mouth infection**
- **the patient might have a fit, is unconscious or confused.**

By armpit

Make sure the skin is dry. Put the thermometer under the arm, the bulb well into the armpit. Fold the arm across the patient's chest. Leave the thermometer in place for three minutes.

Breathing

A complete breath consists of taking in air and then letting it go. The rate of breathing is counted by each rise of the chest. The adult average is 16 to 18 times a minute. A much higher rate may result from bronchitis, viral infection, heart disease, shock and exercise. Babies breathe faster but their breathing can be difficult to detect because it is shallow. Seek medical help if a baby ever has breathing difficulties.

It is best to take the breathing rate when you check the pulse so that you can do it unobtrusively, or do it when the patient is asleep. We can all breathe more quickly or slowly at will and it is difficult not to alter the rate of breathing when you know that your breathing is being watched.

IMPORTANT

Keep medicines safely locked away in a cool dry cupboard.

Never transfer medicines from the original container.

Do not give any medicine if you cannot read the label.

Medicines prescribed for one patient must not be given to anyone else.

Do not use any medicine that has passed the expiry date.

If a doctor changes or stops treatment, dispose of unfinished medicines by flushing them down the toilet.

Medicines by mouth

Pills, tablets and powders

Check the label on the container. Put the right number of tablets in a teaspoon on a saucer and recheck the instructions on the label. Give them to the patient with a glass of water and see that they are taken. Large tablets can be crushed (see right) or divided if the patient finds them difficult to swallow. Capsules and sugar-coated pills should not be crushed or divided. Dissolve powders in water or mix with jam.

Giving medicine to a child

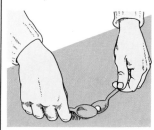

Explain to the child that the medicine is necessary to make him or her well again. Have a glass of fruit juice ready to take away the taste and if the dose has a very unpleasant flavour, try mixing it with honey, jam or yoghurt. Explain that it will not taste so bad this way.

You can make it easier for a small child to swallow tablets by crushing them between two spoons. Mix the powder with honey or jam. Ask the chemist if a liquid medicine is available instead. Be sure to keep all medicines locked up.

Liquid medicines

1 Read the label on the bottle and check that it is the right medicine. Cover the cap with your finger and shake the bottle well a couple of times. Remove the cap. Hold it against your hand with your little finger.

2 Hold the bottle label up so that drips do not fall on the label. Measure out the correct dose into a 5ml spoon; medicine is often supplied with one. Alternatively, measure the dose into a medicine glass.

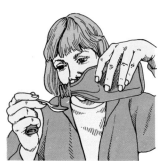

3 Put back the cap of the bottle. Check the dose on the label again. Watch the patient take the dose and offer a drink to take the taste away if this is allowed. Wash the glass or spoon, wipe the bottle and put it away in the medicine cupboard. Never leave medicines by the bedside.

Inhalation

Sometimes an inhalation will relieve a patient of the symptoms of a heavy cold, particularly a blocked nose, and it may help asthma or bronchitis sufferers. Inhalation is the administration of a medicine which is dissolved in very hot water so that the patient breathes in the vapour. The doctor will advise on which inhalant medicine to use.

The method described below is a steam inhalation which is the usual method. Occasionally you may be asked to give an inhalation with a Nelson's inhaler, which is a specially shaped jug. Provide the patient with a sputum cup and tissues to use if they are wanted and offer him or her a mouthwash, a drink of water or fruit juice after the inhalation.

You will need:
- tray
- large jug
- small towel
- large towel
- large bowl
- ½ litre (1 pint) water just off the boil
- inhalant
- 5ml spoon.

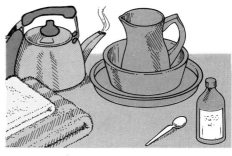

1 The patient must be sitting up well supported. Put petroleum jelly or cream just inside the patient's nostrils so that the inhalant does not irritate them. Put half the hot water in the jug, add the inhalant, then the remaining water. Put the small towel round the base of the jug.

2 Put the jug in the bowl on a tray. Arrange the large towel like a headscarf round the top of the jug. Tell the patient to breathe in through the mouth and out through the nose while the steam rises (about ten minutes).

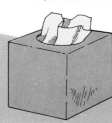

Food and diet

Liquids and food are essential to keep us alive. In the form of a balanced diet they are central to good health and they also give us a great deal of enjoyment. Ideally we should all know what vital nutrients are contained in which foods. This is important when caring for someone who is unwell. Patients may have little appetite for food because of their condition, but they need sustenance to regain their health. Tempt them to eat by making food look attractive. Small helpings of appetising food served at shorter intervals are more appealing than large occasional meals. Encourage patients to drink water.

A balanced diet

We need to eat a balanced diet to:
● maintain a constant body heat
● generate the energy required for movement and the essential functions of the body
● provide for normal body growth
● repair and replace cells.

A balanced diet provides the body with fuel for these functions in the nutrients (goodness) it contains. The importance of these is set out in the chart on the next pages. Most of our food intake is carbohydrate with some fat but it is important to include protein and fibre each day because they cannot be stored in the body. Sufficient liquids are also important.

Our needs vary according to our age, sex and lifestyle. Children need more protein to promote growth, men generally require more to eat than women, people who take a great deal of exercise need more food than someone sitting at a desk all day, or ill in bed. In a cold climate it takes more energy to keep warm, and so a higher intake of food is necessary than in the heat when more liquid is required.

Some people's diets are determined by religious or ethical beliefs. Find out what a patient is happy to eat. Check whether there are any foods which the patient must not eat, either for reasons of belief or because of special medical instructions.

Dietary requirements used to be measured by the calorie but are now sometimes counted as joules (4.18 joules = 1 calorie). Precise amounts have to be calculated only when a patient is on a special diet. The special diets you are most likely to encounter are described on page 57.

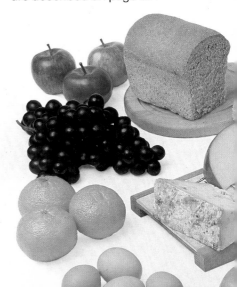

Making meals easier

A deep bowl (below) and light, thick-handled cutlery (left) are best for someone with a weak grip.

A light feeding cup or a glass with an angled straw are easier for helpless patients to drink from.

Convenience foods

Some pre-packaged meals contain mostly stodgy carbohydrate, filling but not sustaining. It is very tempting for someone leading a busy working life or doing the shopping in a hurry to resort to these convenience foods, but they may be low on protein and cannot on their own be considered to provide a balanced diet. Whenever possible food should be fresh, varied and appetising, including some meat, fish, wholemeal bread, fruit and vegetables.

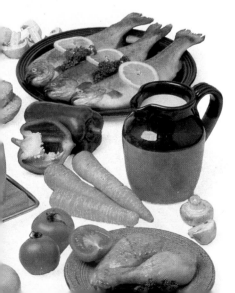

Cutlery and crockery

The physical problems of eating and drinking can make mealtimes very trying for those with a weak grip: arthritis sufferers, elderly and disabled people. Special cutlery and crockery (see above) can overcome these problems.

Common-sense eating

Unless the patient is on a special diet, there are certain common-sense guidelines which can lead to better health in the long term and may involve tactfully breaking down old habits.

● Unless the patient's condition requires easily digestible food, provide plenty of fibre, particularly fruit and vegetables, raw or lightly cooked because over-cooking destroys the vitamins. Patients who eat enough fibre are less likely to be constipated.

● If a patient is overweight, do not offer snacks between meals or an excessive amount of food.

● Limit the amount of fatty foods such as cream, butter and cheese.

● Bake or grill foods; avoid frying.

● Fresh fruit or bran biscuits with cottage cheese make healthier snacks or desserts than sweets or heavy filling puddings.

Dietary essentials

Nutrient	Contained in	Importance
Water	We take in water whenever we drink and at almost all meals. All fluids and most foods contain a high percentage of water.	Water is the most important ingredient of all. It is essential to life. The body is 70% water and nearly all our tissues contain water. It is important to drink enough to replace fluid lost in excretion.
Protein	Meat, fish, poultry, eggs, milk, nuts, peas, beans, cereals, honey.	An essential part of the daily diet because the body cannot store protein. It is essential for cell repair and replacement, so is particularly important after injury or during illness. Protein is vital to normal growth and so to children and women who are pregnant or breast-feeding.
Carbohydrates	Some root vegetables such as potatoes and parsnips, bread, pasta, rice, cereals, fruit sugar, sugar and all foods sweetened by it (cakes, icecreams, sweets and jams, for example).	Carbohydrates are essential fuel foods. The body derives glucose for immediate energy from sugars and starches, but if too much carbohydrate is eaten, the body converts it into fat.
Fats	Milk, butter, margarine, cheese, cream, cooking fat, olive oil, fish oils, meat fat, egg yolk.	Fats provide long-term energy and warmth. We usually eat more fatty foods in cold weather but some "hot weather" foods like icecream have a high fat content. Excessive intake of fats is bad for the heart and blood vessels.
Fibre (roughage) 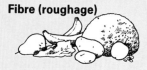	Wholemeal bread, bran, bran cereals, unrefined flour, fresh fruit, vegetables, lentils.	Although our bodies cannot absorb fibre, it is very important for digestion and excretion.

Nutrient	Contained in	Importance
Mineral salts particularly iron	Milk, liver, eggs, green or yellow vegetables (such as spinach, Brussels sprouts and celery), fish, baked beans.	Mineral salts are needed only in small amounts and a balanced diet provides these. Iron is the element most commonly lacking in the right amount particularly in pregnant women, for whom iron tablets are often prescribed.
Vitamin A	Milk, liver, fish liver oils, eggs, cheese, butter. Vitamin A is also made by the body from yellow fruits such as apricots and tomatoes and carrots.	Vitamin A promotes growth and provides defence against infection. It is essential to good sight, but it is possible to take too much vitamin A.
B group of vitamins	Many meats particularly liver, unprocessed cereal, yeast, green vegetables, milk and eggs.	These vitamins help break down food for energy and produce red blood cells. They help in brain, nerve and muscle functions. Lack of B vitamins causes problems with skin, the nervous system and digestion.
Vitamin C	Fresh fruit, particularly citrus fruit, some green vegetables.	Vitamin C helps the body's healing power and so fights infection. It is important in growth and in our response to stress. Because the body cannot store it, we need to have some daily.
Vitamin D	Eggs, butter and fish (particularly fish-liver oils). It is also made by the body when the skin is exposed to sunlight.	Vitamin D in moderate amounts is necessary for good bone development. Both the lack of it and excess cause problems.
Vitamin E	Milk, eggs, cereals, liver, wheatgerm.	Vitamin E helps to keep cells healthy.

Food presentation

Meals should always be anticipated with pleasure. Time passes slowly for someone in bed and meals help to break up the day. Always find out what a patient is allowed to eat and ask if there is anything he or she really dislikes. Establish whether the patient can cut up food or needs help.

Patients should have the opportunity to use the lavatory, commode or urinal and to wash their hands before each meal. Offer as much help as patients need and see that they are in a comfortable position in bed or sitting up well supported in a chair before you bring in the food.

To provide a meal on a tray

See that everything needed is attractively laid out on a clean tray. Take care not to overfill containers of drink or soup or they will slop. Heat hot dishes thoroughly, serving them on hot plates. If there are several courses, do not take in everything at once. Allow enough time for the patient to eat but when he or she has finished the meal take the tray from the room.

Meals for helpless patients

Patients who cannot manage their own meals will need your help. This is an extremely important part of your care. Always sit by the patient's side, within easy reach so that both of you feel comfortable. It is important to be on the unaffected side of a stroke patient. Protect the patient and the bedclothes. Take trouble with presentation of meals so that the food appears appetising. Offer small mouthfuls, allowing the patient time to chew properly and swallow. Remember to give the patient enough to drink.

Patients without teeth

Those patients who do not have their own teeth or dentures may need their food liquidised or put through a mincer, sieve or food processor because chewing may be uncomfortable for them. If a semi-solid diet has been ordered, you will be told what to give.

Blind patients

Those who cannot see are usually able to feed themselves. Find out first how your patient likes meals served so you can help without infringing on his or her independence. Explain how the food is arranged on the plate like a clockface: vegetables at 3 o'clock, chicken at 7 o'clock and so on. If the patient requires feeding, agree on a squeeze on the shoulder or a light tap on the hand to indicate that the next mouthful is ready, so that you can hold a normal uninterrupted conversation.

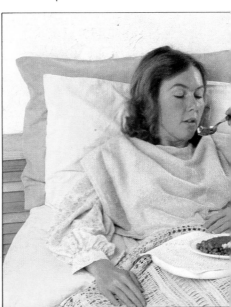

Special diets

What a patient can eat may be determined by the nature of the illness. A doctor or dietician will in some instances plan out a specific diet which must be followed in detail. Broad guidelines are sometimes sufficient, setting down the foods that are permitted and those that must be avoided, giving some freedom of choice. When you are looking after someone, your aim is always to provide food which is as nutritious and interesting as possible within any set limits.

Encourage a child on a strict diet by offering food on bright plates and drinks through striped or curly straws.

Light diets

Foods that are easily digestible are the basis of a light diet: fish, white meat, eggs, milk, bread and butter, puréed fruit and small quantities of vegetables and fruit juice.

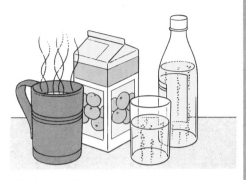

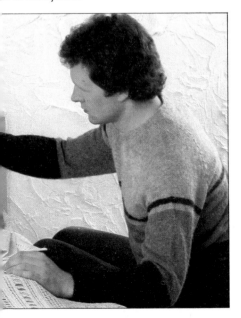

Fluids only

An adult patient will need not less than 3 litres (5 pints) of fluid daily. Remember that since the average cup holds 150ml (5 oz) this means about 20 cups of liquid each day. A proportion of this ought to be milk, yoghurt, jelly or soups. Flavourings such as coffee, cocoa and Horlicks can be added, if the patient wishes. A protein supplement such as Complan is often given with a fluids-only diet.

Diabetes

Diet is important in the control of this disease in which the patient's body cannot store glucose. He or she is usually given guidelines limiting the carbohydrate intake. It is very important to follow these if you are looking after a patient with diabetes.

Low-calorie diet

This is a diet prescribed for someone who is overweight. Carbohydrates and fats are strictly limited. These are replaced by fruits, salads and vegetables. Overweight people are more likely to suffer from a variety of ailments. The purpose of the low-calorie diet is both to reduce the patient's weight and to lead him or her into new eating habits and a healthier life.

Feeding a baby

After birth a woman's breasts fill with milk for the baby. Breast milk is best for the baby physically but only if breast-feeding suits the mother emotionally. The well-being of the baby and the happiness of the mother are both important and no-one should make her feel guilty or embarrassed whether she decides to breast-feed or bottle-feed the baby. Expert advice on how to feed a new baby is available from a midwife, health visitor or from classes the mother can attend before the birth.

Teaching a baby to feed

A new baby has to learn that the answer to hunger is food, which comes from the nipple or teat. The hungry baby will instinctively turn towards a gentle touch or stroking on the cheek, pursing the lips ready to suck. It may take the baby and mother a few weeks to establish feeding happily.

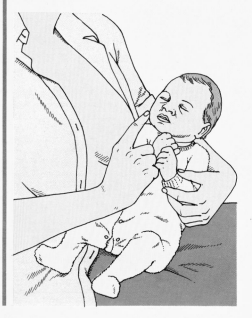

When to feed

New babies rarely want to feed by routine, so fixed feeding times may not be possible. Feeding on demand (when the baby wants to) probably suits both the baby and mother better. The baby does not need to cry hungrily until it is "time" for a feed or be woken from sleep, but is fed whenever he or she is hungry. A newborn baby needs feeding very often, perhaps every two hours to begin with. By the age of two months this will have eased to every three or four hours, but the baby's demands may be irregular. At least one feed at night will be necessary for the first six weeks and generally for several months. The baby will gradually need less at night. The parents and anyone helping with the baby will eventually have unbroken nights' sleep again, but in the meantime that night feed is very important.

Wind and colic

Most babies take in some air when crying or feeding. This is known as getting wind. Their sucking is not very strong in the first months and they may gulp in air with the milk. In case wind causes discomfort, pause mid-feed or at the end of the feed, put the baby against your shoulder and rub his or her back gently. A little milk may come up with the air.

Sometimes a baby is particularly distressed at the same time every evening. He or she cries a great deal and curls up, seeming to have tummy pains. The trouble may be colic. Little is known about it, but it is quite common, and usually ceases when the baby is three months old. The health visitor or doctor may be able to help.

Breast-feeding

Breast milk is perfect for babies. It is instantly available, at the right temperature, and needs no special storage, mixing or sterilisation.

Many women worry because their milk looks watery compared to cows' milk, but it has a high protein content and all the carbohydrates, vitamins and minerals the baby needs. It is easy for the baby to digest and contains antibodies that give some protection against illness.

The mother needs to eat a healthy protein-rich diet while she is feeding her baby (see page 54). She will probably find it easier to feed her baby if she is given quiet and privacy, at least in the first weeks.

How much and how long

Some mothers wonder if a baby is getting the right amount of milk. It is not easy to tell exactly how much a baby has taken when breast-feeding. But it is not possible to over-feed a breast-fed baby and under-feeding is rare. A mother can soon tell if the baby is satisfied and has taken enough.

How long the baby will want to feed for will vary but up to ten minutes sucking at each breast is usually enough. Some babies obtain all they want within the first five minutes, others take much longer. It is best to start each feed on the alternate breast.

Common anxieties

Many mothers are anxious about breast-feeding. They worry about having enough milk and whether the baby will flourish on it. Most problems are short-lived, and after the first few days the mother's supply adapts to the needs of her baby. Expert advice is always available from the health visitor or family doctor.

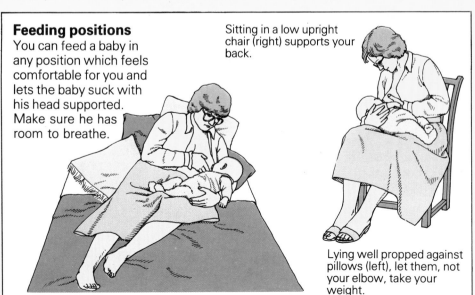

Feeding positions
You can feed a baby in any position which feels comfortable for you and lets the baby suck with his head supported. Make sure he has room to breathe.

Sitting in a low upright chair (right) supports your back.

Lying well propped against pillows (left), let them, not your elbow, take your weight.

Bottle~feeding

There are occasionally times when a mother is unable to breast-feed her baby or is really not happy about the idea of doing so. Then of course bottle-feeding will be necessary and the baby will thrive if proper care is taken. Always wash your hands before preparing feeds or giving them.

Formula milk

The milk usually chosen to bottle-feed a baby is made up from dried cows' milk, specially adapted for babies to make it resemble human milk as nearly as possible. *It is dangerous to give a small baby ordinary cows' milk.* Milk powder can be bought from most food shops, child health clinics or chemists. Always ask if the kind you are buying is safe for babies. Baby milk can also be bought as a liquid formula, but it may not be available everywhere.

Bottles and teats

The baby feeds by sucking through a rubber teat shaped like a human nipple. Teats should allow milk out of an upturned bottle at the rate of several drops a second.

Bottles are made of glass or plastic and may be disposable. Usually the volume measurements are marked up the side so you can make up feeds accurately and also tell how much a baby has taken when feeding. Bottles should have no lips or sharp corners so that they are easy to clean.

Sterilising feeding equipment

All bottles, teats and equipment must be sterile before use. You must maintain strict standards of cleanliness. Wash your hands before you handle feeding equipment. Bottles, teats, spoons, knives and jugs must all be

---

Making up feeds

Put all equipment on a clear clean surface. Follow the instructions on the container exactly. *Liquid formulas*: wash the top and sterilise it by pouring boiling water over before opening it.

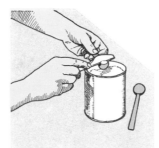 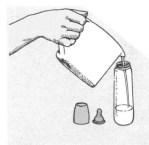

1 *Powder formulas*: Wash your hands. Boil water and let it cool to hand heat. Remove equipment from the sterilising unit. Pour the right amount of boiled warm water into the jug. Check it at eye level.

2 Scoop out the milk powder. Level off measures with a knife blade without packing it down in any way. Add it to the jug and stir the mixture thoroughly so that the powder dissolves completely.

3 Fill the bottles to the right level, checking the amount carefully. Screw on the teats upside down and put the bottles in the fridge. Even in the fridge feeds should be kept for only one day.

sterilised. All bottles and teats should be thoroughly rinsed in cold water after use, then washed in warm water with washing up liquid and rinsed again. Use a bottle brush because it enables you to clean all surfaces properly.

The best way of sterilising them is to submerge them in a special sterilising container filled with sterile solution. The equipment must be completely covered and remain in the solution for the right time (see the manufacturer's instructions given with the sterilising agent). It is a good idea to leave things in solution until they are needed so that there is no possibility of any bacteria infecting them.

Giving a bottle feed

If you are giving a bottle-feed to someone else's baby always ask for any special instructions they may have about making up and giving the feed. Remove the bottle from the fridge and put it in a container of hot water (not boiling). Shake a few drops of milk on to the back of your hand or your wrist. It should be warm not hot. Always hold the bottle pointing downwards so that the teat is full of milk, not air and milk. If the baby does not take the full bottle, any left-over milk must be thrown away, *never* kept for a later feed.

Getting comfortable for the feed is just as important as for breast-feeding and the baby also needs to feel close and secure. The baby's mother should feed him or her as much as possible.

Weaning

This is the term used for the gradual introduction of solid food into the baby's diet. The baby can obtain all the nutrients needed from milk up to the age of four months or more and is not able to digest solid foods until about that age.

Try out new foods in tiny quantities. Only offer soft foods that can be swallowed without chewing. These could include puréed fruit and vegetables, baby cereals, gravy, finely minced meat and soups. There are many kinds of brand-name baby foods available which are convenient, but fresh foods are better because you can control the content. Do not add salt or sugar. Avoid oily or spicy foods and excessive fibre. Watch the baby carefully in case an upset digestion results in diarrhoea (see page 39). If the baby refuses any food do not try it again for three or four days. The changeover from milk to solid foods is usually a slow process and may take up to six months or so.

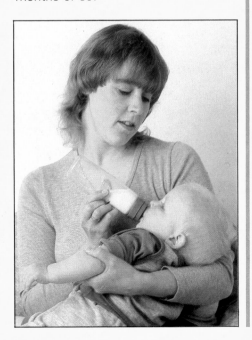

Injuries

There may be times when you have to care for someone with an injury, perhaps by providing first aid when it happens or by nursing the patient afterwards. The commonest injuries you might encounter are wounds, bruises, sprained joints, strained muscles, burns and scalds. Injuries must be kept clean and may need to be covered and supported while the healing process takes place.

Dressings and bandages

It is easier to respond to any injuries quickly and efficiently if there is an adequate medicine cupboard or first-aid kit. The equipment must remain clean and dry, so it should ideally be kept somewhere other than in the bathroom in case it is affected by steam and well out of the reach of children. Label the container of your medical equipment clearly so you or anyone else can

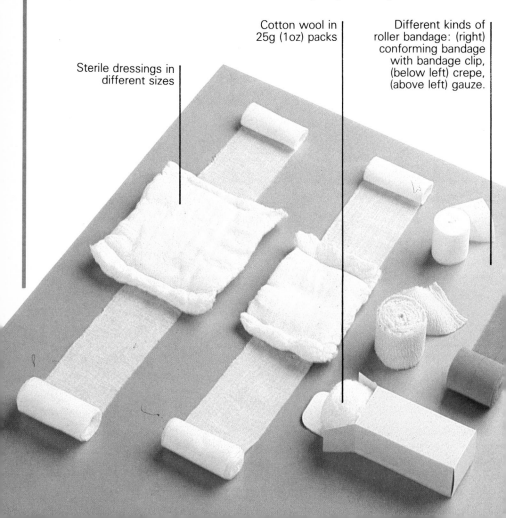

Cotton wool in 25g (1oz) packs

Different kinds of roller bandage: (right) conforming bandage with bandage clip, (below left) crepe, (above left) gauze.

Sterile dressings in different sizes

identify it immediately it is needed. The equipment you might need for cleaning and dressing wounds is shown in the photograph below.

There are two main types of dressing and two main types of bandage. *Sterile dressings* are used for large or serious wounds and consist of a thick pad of gauze and cotton wool attached to a roller bandage. They are sealed in sterile packets which should only be opened just before use. *Adhesive dressings* (plasters) are absorbent gauze pads with an adhesive, preferably water-repellent, backing. They are individually wrapped. Both kinds of dressing are available in different sizes and the size used should extend well beyond the area of the wound.

A *triangular bandage* is a large triangular piece of material which is most useful as a sling. There should be one in any home medical kit. *Roller bandages* are effective in holding a dressing in place and providing support for a sprain or strain. It is useful to have several roller bandages.

Gauze pads

Adhesive strapping

Safety pins in different sizes

Triangular bandage

Adhesive dressings in different sizes

Scissors

Tweezers

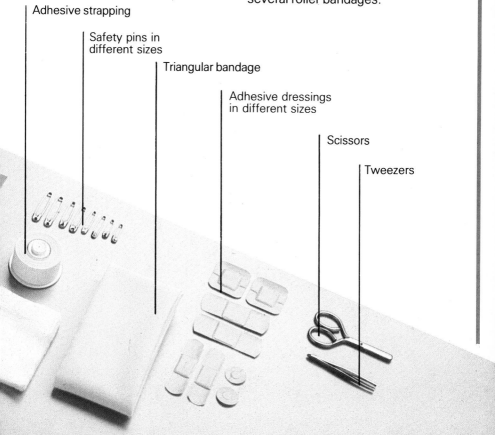

Caring for wounds

This must be done in a spotlessly clean manner to prevent the entry of germs. Wash any equipment and your hands before you start. Germs are micro-organisms, which are present in all kinds of dirt, and if they enter a wound can multiply fast causing infection.

When you are dressing a wound, do not disturb the air unnecessarily in case dust or bacteria settle on the wound. Close the windows and door to avoid draughts. Sit the patient down and explain what you are about to do, then keep talking to a minimum while the wound is exposed to avoid breathing over it. Never cough or sneeze over an wound. If the condition of a wound causes concern, consult a doctor.

Large wounds

Your nursing care of these will probably be limited to changing dressings, either as an aid to a district nurse (who will bring sterile equipment) or on your own. A plug or clot forms across the surface of a wound to stop bleeding. It is important to be gentle in caring for the wound or you may disturb a clot and cause further bleeding. If a dressing is stuck, do not attempt to remove it — the district nurse or doctor will do this.

Small cuts and grazes

These are the commonest injuries at home and children are the most likely sufferers. A graze happens when the top layers of skin are scraped off in a sliding fall, exposing an area of raw tender skin. Cuddle and comfort a child after a graze. Small cuts and grazes often ooze blood and may be dirty. Clean them thoroughly as soon as possible after the injury.

To clean a wound you will need:

- soap and water
- cotton wool, gauze swabs or antiseptic wipes
- bag for soiled swabs
- absorbent kitchen paper
- appropriate dressing.

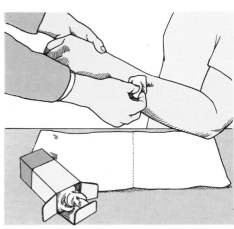

Wash your hands. Gather your equipment on to a clean covered surface. If the wound is dirty, rinse it under cold running water if possible. Then gently clean around it with soap and water, using cotton wool, gauze swabs or anti-septic wipes. Work from the centre of the wound outwards and take a new swab for each stroke. If the wound is a graze, dab it very gently. You can temporarily cover the wound with white kitchen paper if necessary. Apply an adhesive dressing to a small wound and a sterile dressing to a larger one. Make sure the pad will extend beyond the wound.

Serious wounds should be seen by a doctor. If there is anything stuck in a wound, do not try to remove it; such wounds should be seen by a doctor as soon as possible.

Applying a sterile dressing

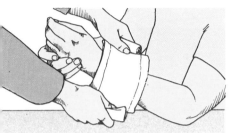

1 Unwind the short end of the sterile dressing and unfold the pad, taking care not to touch the surface that will be against the wound. Gently place the pad, gauze-side down, on the wound.

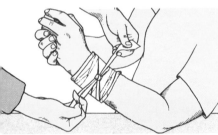

2 Wind the short end once round the limb and the dressing. Then bandage (see page 66) over the pad with the rest of the roll. Tie the ends together over the pad in a reef knot (see page 68).

Applying an adhesive dressing

1 Take the dressing out of its wrapping and hold it gauze-side down by the protective strips. Peel back these strips to expose the gauze but do not remove them completely. Without touching the gauze, place the dressing over the wound.

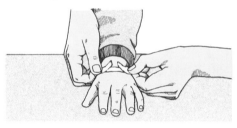

2 Gently pull off the protective strip and press down the edges.

3 If you need to remove the dressing, pull it off gently but firmly, after a bath when it will come off easily.

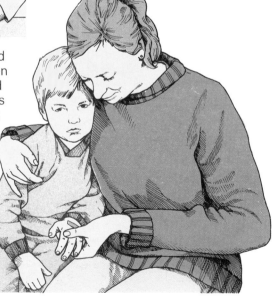

Calming the patient
A child may feel frightened and bewildered by the pain of a graze or the sight of blood. Gently comfort him and explain that a plaster helps to keep dirt out.

Roller bandages

These are made of cotton, crepe, muslin, flannel or special paper. The right widths for bandaging arms or legs, the areas you are most likely to deal with, are 5–7cm (2–3in). The roll is usually about 5m (5yd) long.

The aim of a roller bandage is to hold a dressing in place or to provide support for an injury such as a sprain or strain. Apply a bandage with even pressure. If it is too tight, it will reduce the blood flow to the area. Check that it is not too tight immediately after applying the bandage and ten minutes after. If the patient's skin is pale and cold or if finger or toenails go blue, re-apply the bandage immediately.

The bandage should be rolled tightly. Sit the patient down and support the injured part. Stand in front of the patient on the injured side. If the wound is on part of the body of even size such as a forearm, use the simple spiral pattern shown below. Use the figure-of-eight pattern for awkward areas such as hands and feet.

Spiral pattern

1 Work from below upwards and from the inside to the outside. Hold the bandage, roll uppermost, and secure the end by making a firm turn round below the area of the wound or injury.

2 Working up the limb make a series of spiral turns round the limb with the bandage. With each turn cover two-thirds of the previous one, keeping an even pressure on the bandage.

3 Make a straight turn above the dressing. Fold under the end. Fasten it with a safety pin or bandage clip (see inset) or tie it (see opposite). Make sure the bandage is not too tight.

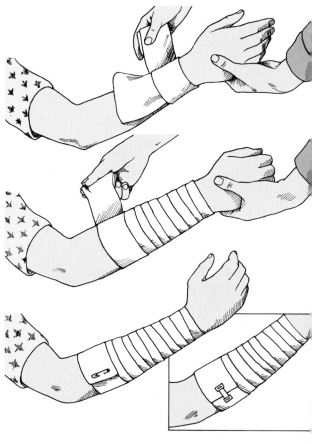

Securing a bandage

Fasten the end of a bandage with a safety pin, adhesive tape or special bandage clips. If the patient is a child or no fastenings are available, the bandage can be tied. Leave at least 15cm (6in) of the bandage free, or enough to go round the affected area, cut it down the middle and tie a knot at the bottom. Tie off round the limb with a reef knot (see page 69).

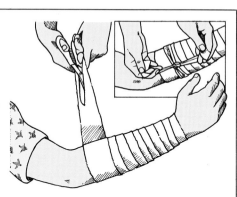

Figure-of-eight

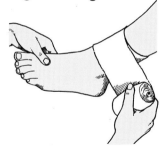 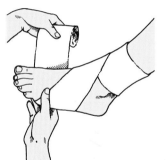 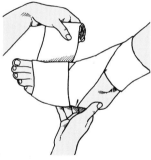

1 Raise and support the foot and make one straight turn around the ankle to secure the bandage.

2 Take the bandage across the top of the foot towards the little toe, under the foot and up by the base of the big toe.

3 Bring the bandage across the top of the foot to the little toe. Make another turn under the base of the toes.

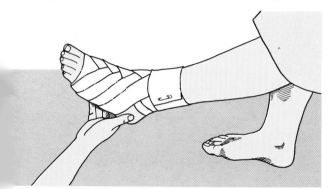

4 Take the bandage across the top of the foot and round behind the ankle. Continue making figure-of-eight turns until the foot is covered. Finish off with a straight turn round the ankle and secure the end. If the patient's toes become cold or the nails blue, re-apply the bandage.

Applying an arm sling

Triangular bandages can be used as slings to support an injured hand, arm or wrist. Healing is promoted because any wound heals faster if it is rested. If there is no triangular bandage available, you can make one by cutting diagonally across a 1m (1yd) square of firmly woven fabric such as linen or calico, or use a large scarf folded in half diagonally. Before applying an arm sling, sit the patient down. Ask him or her to support the injured limb with the hand; be prepared to help. Fold in a narrow hem along the base of the triangular bandage.

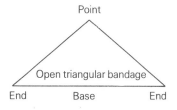

Point

Open triangular bandage

End   Base   End

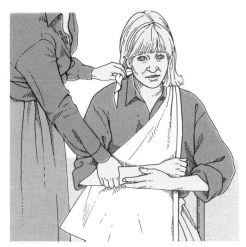

1 Use the space between chest and elbow to ease the bandage gently into place, leaving the point beyond the elbow. Take the top end round the patient's neck. Let the base of the bandage hang down the body.

Reef knots

A reef knot is the correct knot to use to secure the ends of bandages because it does not slip, it lies flat and so is comfortable for the patient and it is easy to unfasten. The ends can be neatly tucked under, but do make sure that no part of the knot presses on the patient. If it might do so, put a soft pad of material or cotton wool underneath the reef knot.

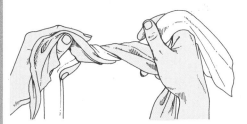

1 Hold one end of the bandage in each hand. Take the right end over the left and pass it underneath.

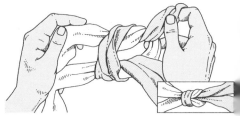

2 Bring what is now the left end up, over the right and under it again. Pull the knot tight and tuck the ends in.

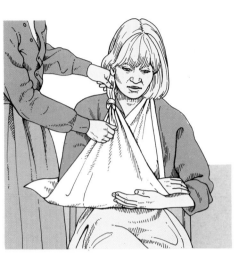

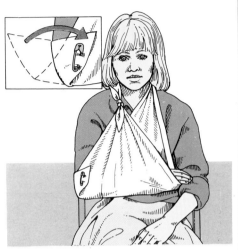

2 Bring the bottom end of the bandage up over the arm to the neck. Make a reef knot (see below) to tie off the ends of the bandage on the injured side in the hollow above the collar bone.

3 Tuck the excess bandage behind the elbow (see inset). Bring the point forward and secure it in the front with a safety pin. Check that the patient's circulation is not affected. If it is, re-apply the sling.

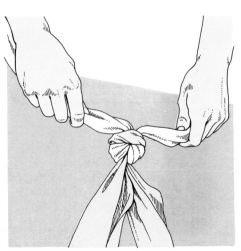

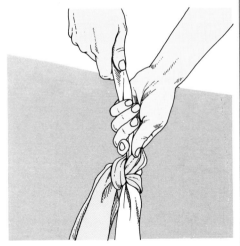

3 When you need to untie the knot take hold of one pair of bandage ends close to the knot and pull them.

4 You can now slip the knot apart easily by sliding one end of the bandage off the other.

Inflammation

This is the body's response to infection in a wound or to damaged tissue. The inflamed area becomes swollen, red and hot and may be very painful. The patient sometimes has difficulty using the part and may develop a raised temperature and increased pulse rate. The best ways to offer relief are to apply a cold compress or a hot poultice. As a rule, cold is used to treat a recent injury, heat an older one but heat may localise and draw out infection.

Cold compresses

These are cold pads applied to the skin to cool it down. They are used to minimise the swelling and pain of injuries such as bruising and strained joints. They reduce the blood flow in the area and are most effective if they are applied as soon as possible after injury. However, treatment is some-times repeated under instruction from a district nurse or doctor. There are several methods of making a cold com-press. Compresses are usually left in place for at least 20 minutes.

Hot poultices

These are soft semi-liquid packs which are applied to the skin to transfer heat. The heat stops infection spreading by increasing the flow of blood in the area. Hot poultices are usually applied on the instructions of a district nurse or doctor; never apply one to a recent injury. Kaolin, a clay with medicated oils, makes a good poultice because it holds heat well. It can be bought in tins or as ready-made poultices, which are not as widely available but are much simpler to use. A covered hot water bottle can be used if the injury or infection is not severe.

Cold water packs

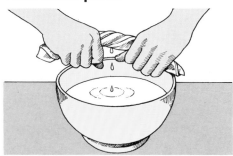

Soak a face flannel, thin towel or pad of cotton wool in very cold or iced water. Wring it out so that it stops dripping, holding it by the ends to avoid warming it. Fold it to the right size and place it on the affected area which should be well supported. Replace the pack every ten minutes with a new one or drip very cold water on to the original pack so that it continues to cool.

Ice packs

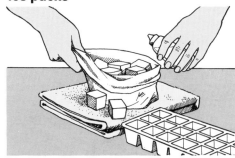

Fill a plastic bag up to two-thirds full of ice. Either crush the ice first or add a little salt to make the ice melt faster. Squeeze out the air and seal the bag with a tie or wire closure. Wrap it in a thin towel and place it on the area. The patient should be sitting comfortably with the injury well supported while the compress is in place.

Ready-made poultices

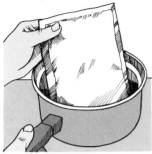

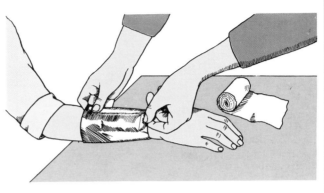

1 Apply some petroleum jelly or a little olive oil to the affected area. Put the poultice sachet foil-side up in a saucepan and pour boiling water over it. Leave it for 40 seconds. Remove the sachet and take off the plastic cover.

2 Test the heat first to make sure it will not burn. Place the poultice on the skin and secure it with a bandage (see pages 66–67). Leave the poultice in place for up to 12 hours or for as long as the nurse or doctor has recommended.

Note This kind of poultice can be used as a cold compress by placing it in an ice compartment or deep freeze for an hour. Do not remove the cover. Wrap the compress in a thin towel and put it on the skin. Leave it in place for 20 minutes.

Making a poultice

If you cannot buy a pre-pared poultice, use a tin of kaolin. Loosen the lid before putting the tin in boiling water, which should not cover the top. When the kaolin is hot, spread it evenly on a piece of clean old linen. Test the heat on your arm to make sure that it will not burn the patient. Apply the poultice, cover with cotton wool and bandage it in position.

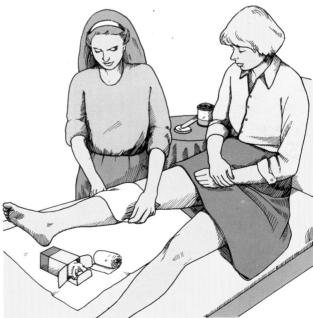

Infectious diseases

A number of diseases which are communicated from person to person are quite common. The ones shown on the lower part of the chart opposite are usually thought of as "childhood" diseases. Babies are at first protected by the immunity (resistance) they inherit from their mothers but this wears off. The diseases are common and very infectious so a child will certainly be exposed to some of them at some stage and may develop an illness the first time he or she is in contact with someone who has it. The germs which cause infection are spread on the air, by dust, insects, infected food, other infected objects such as books and linen and by other people. With most of these diseases there is a known period of time, called the incubation period, between becoming infected and the symptoms appearing.

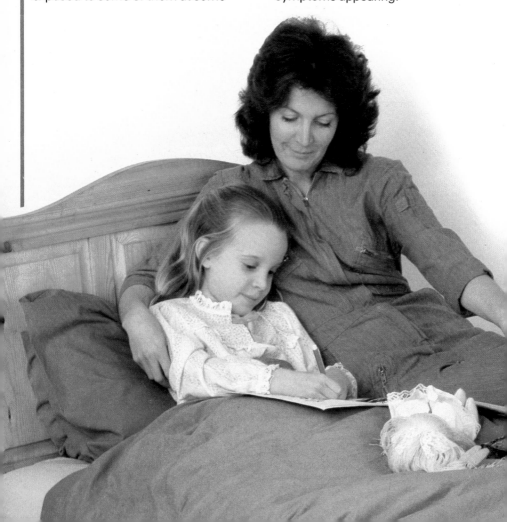

Disease	Incubation period	Symptoms
Influenza (flu)	2–3 days	Rise of temperature, sore throat, runny nose, cough, hoarse voice, headache, aching joints.
Gastroenteritis	Varies considerably	Diarrhoea, vomiting, tummy pains.
Chickenpox	14–21 days	Rise of temperature. Dark red itchy clusters of spots which appear over a period of several days.
German measles	10–14 days	Slightly raised temperature, rash starting behind the ears spreading to face and body.
Measles	11–21 days	Runny nose, cough, sore eyes, raised temperature, white spots in the mouth, blotchy red rash behind ears spreading to the face and the body.
Mumps	17–21 days	Swelling and pain in glands at side of face, stiff neck and jaw, earache, rise of temperature.
Whooping cough	6–18 days	Slight rise of temperature, coughing in spasms which end with a gasping "whoop".

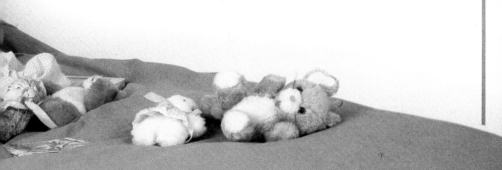

Nursing care

How you care for the patient will depend on how ill he or she feels and on the nature of the infection. An adult with an acute attack of mumps will feel really ill and might need special nursing care, a child with a mild infection of German measles may just feel a bit off colour. If a young baby catches gastro-enteritis, he or she might be very ill and need hospital care.

Most children with infectious diseases will need a lot of love and attention. A child does not always need to stay in bed but should have enough rest and keep warm. The patient may not want to eat much food for several days but should be encouraged to drink as much liquid as possible. Offer plenty of water and ask the doctor what other fluids are allowed. This is particularly important if the illness is accompanied by any sickness or diarrhoea. The doctor may recommend a particular amount of liquid each day.

If the patient's temperature is above 39.5°C (103°F), you can lower it by sponging down. This is done in much the same way as giving a bed bath (see page 30). Lay the patient down on a couple of towels and sponge his or her body with luke-warm water. Check the temperature every 10 minutes and stop when it is lower by one degree. Dry the skin and let the patient stay dressed in cotton or in bed covered with a sheet in a warm but well-aired room. Make sure that the patient does not get chilled.

If the patient has an itchy rash, soothe it with the prescribed lotion applied with cotton wool and explain to a child that the spots will hurt more and last longer if they are scratched.

Treating a rash
The rash that accompanies most infectious diseases may be very itchy. The doctor may advise using a soothing lotion.

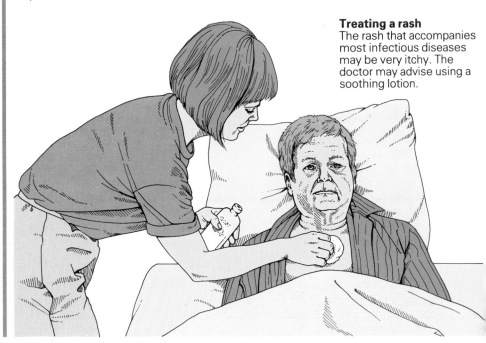

Controlling infection

Schools and other institutions used to insist that a child with an infectious disease was kept away to prevent the spread of infection. However, a disease is most infectious at the end of the incubation period and as the symptoms appear, when it may not have been diagnosed. It is now thought that there is little advantage in isolating the patient at home. It may be better for a child to catch an infection when young and get it over with because some childhood diseases can make an older patient very ill. The doctor or district nurse will tell you whether to allow visitors and if you need to take any particular precautions. Efficient hygiene does help to restrict the spread, so be prompt and careful in clearing away bedpans, commodes and food left-overs. Always wash your hands after caring for the patient so that you do not transmit germs.

Immunity

Not everyone who is in contact with an infectious disease will necessarily develop the illness. Their bodies may be able to fight off the infection if they are in good general health, have been exposed to the disease before or have been immunised. This is a form of protection that can be offered against certain diseases. A person is given, usually by injection, a weakened version of the germs that cause a particular disease. He or she does not become ill but the body's defences are brought into action against the germs and stay active for many years.

Injections against measles and whooping cough are usually offered in a baby's second year. Children are often routinely injected against other less

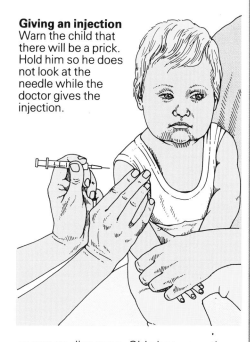

Giving an injection
Warn the child that there will be a prick. Hold him so he does not look at the needle while the doctor gives the injection.

common diseases. Girls between the ages of 11 and 14 should be injected against German measles, to give them immunity before they consider having a child, because if a woman develops German measles early in pregnancy, the infection may damage the unborn child. Community nurses and doctors are always willing to give advice about immunisation.

There has been much discussion about immunisation in recent years. Very occasionally a child becomes seriously ill after an injection, but the risk from the injection is generally held to be much less than the risk of the disease itself. It is probably best for the individual child to be immunised and it is certainly better for the community. Outbreaks of infectious diseases are rare in areas where the rate of immunisation is high.

Special nursing

People home from hospital, the elderly and patients with particular mental or physical handicaps need especially thoughtful care. They may be confused by loss of muscle power or mental agility. They may be tired, weak or depressed. Your understanding, practical care and emotional support can do much to boost their morale and bolster their fragile independence.

Find out how much activity a patient can cope with and what kind, how much rest he or she needs and if any medicines have been prescribed. You and anyone else concerned with the patient's care should be aiming to enable him or her to lead as full and normal a life as possible.

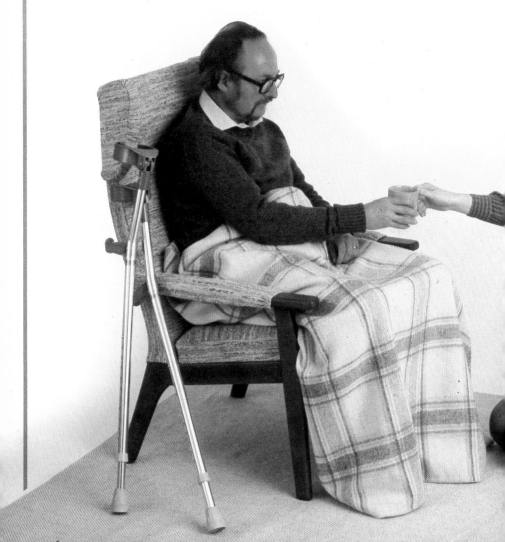

Patients home from hospital

Leaving hospital can make the patient exhausted. The excitement of coming home and the return to near normality may encourage the patient to try to do everything regardless of his or her condition. Most patients are more tired and weak than they expect to be.

Encourage members of the patient's family to provide as much practical help as they can. If you or they can carry out necessary tasks such as food shopping and preparing meals, the patient's limited energy can go towards recovery. What a patient can cope with varies with his or her condition. Someone who has had an operation on the tummy will not be able to do any lifting or carrying. A new mother will be so taken up with caring for her baby that she will have little time for household chores. She is bound to be tired, anxious and in need of any available help. If she becomes worried about the baby's health, or depressed, contact the health visitor or doctor right away. A child may need gently easing back into everyday life with a lot of attention and loving. Children often feel very insecure and periods of bed-wetting and clinging behaviour may follow.

Your priorities are to ensure that the patient gets enough sleep, to provide a healthy diet with sufficient liquid, to provide a listening ear and to encourage the patient to take exercise. The doctor or district nurse will give guidance about what kind of exercise is possible.

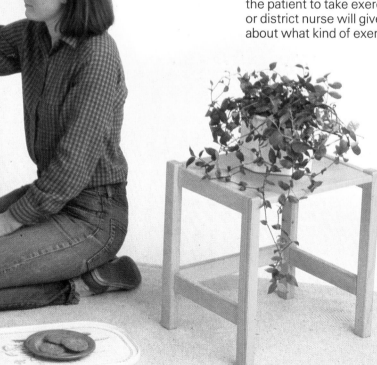

Nursing the elderly

Elderly people often have more health worries as their bodies gradually start to function less well. There are some specific problems such as sleeplessness, breathing difficulties, arthritis and rheumatism that are more common amongst the elderly.

Hypothermia

This is a condition that develops if the body temperature drops below 35°C (95°F), usually due to sitting for a long time in an unheated or poorly heated room. Because of this it is very important for old people to keep warm. Encourage them to install and use adequate heating and if they are worried about not being able to afford it, urge them to seek help from the Social Security Department. Suggest that an elderly person wears extra warm light clothing and see that he or she has a little regular exercise if possible, even if it consists only of walking round at home. Check that the

patient's diet is healthy and includes some hot drinks. If someone is not very mobile, perhaps you could leave a vacuum flask filled with a hot drink within reach.

If you ever find an elderly person very pale, with a very cold skin, intense shivering and slurred speech, suspect hypothermia. Check the pulse and breathing. If the pulse is slow and weak and breathing is slow and shallow, send for the doctor or an ambulance. Wrap the patient loosely in a blanket, keep him or her quiet and warm the room if possible. Give warm drinks but *do not* use a hot water bottle or electric blanket as it will draw heat out of the patient's body.

Sleeplessness

Older people need less sleep. Some elderly people manage quite happily on only several hours of sleep a night, but many others worry when they lie awake. They believe that they need

Lifting
Elderly people should be careful to avoid muscle injury because their muscles heal more slowly. When picking up a heavy weight, bend from the knees rather than from the waist.

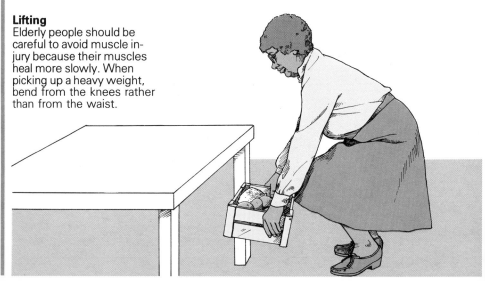

more sleep than they are getting, but often the more they worry the less likely they are to be able to drop off. If you are caring for someone who is unusually wakeful and unhappy about it, there are a number of ways you can help him or her:

● make sure that he or she is comfortable in bed, that the sheets are smooth and the room is warm and aired
● some of the simple aids to comfort shown on page 24 might help
● find out the person's habits — if he or she likes a tot of alcohol or a late evening snack, try to provide it
● suggest a warm bath in the evening
● suggest that stimulants like coffee are avoided in the evening; hot milk drinks or herb teas are more relaxing
● if the patient has breathing problems, he or she is more likely to be able to sleep if there are plenty of well-puffed up pillows (see page 24)
● listen to the patient's anxieties and be as comforting as possible.

Adapting to old age

Encourage elderly people to make life as easy for themselves as possible. There are many kinds of aids and equipment available to help people with limited mobility (see pages 83–85).

Few old people have the energy for hectic exercise but playing gentler sports such as golf, bowls or croquet will help them keep fit and provide welcome company.

Loneliness is one of the greatest problems for the elderly. Any care you give will be valuable because of your friendship and company as much as for the help you are able to offer. Someone coping with a new disability, with grief, sleeplessness or pain may really need to talk out his or her feelings and you should make time to listen and be supportive. An elderly person may not be able to get up after a fall, go shopping or hear the telephone. If you know someone like this, be a good friend or neighbour. Drop by and help regularly.

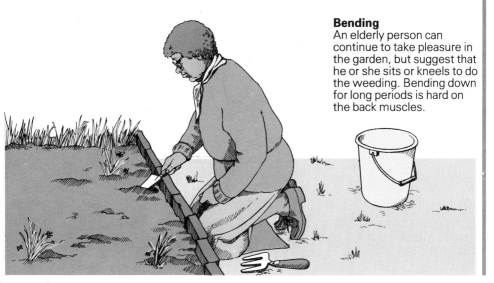

Bending
An elderly person can continue to take pleasure in the garden, but suggest that he or she sits or kneels to do the weeding. Bending down for long periods is hard on the back muscles.

Handicapped children

Babies are born knowing nothing about the world. Normally they learn very quickly about their surroundings, themselves and other people. Curiosity leads them to touch, taste and explore anything within reach. As the skills involved in movement and language are mastered, the young child's experience grows considerably. If all of this takes place within a loving family, the child's development is usually normal.

The development of handicap

A child is said to be physically handicapped if his body has suffered some permanent damage, perhaps becoming unable to see (blind) or hear (deaf) or losing the power of movement. If the damage is to the brain, the child may be mentally handicapped. Mental and physical development are very closely linked in the first couple of years. If a child is physically unable to explore his or her surroundings because of a handicap, that child may appear retarded simply because the means of learning have been limited. A mentally retarded child might seem physically handicapped because he or she is slow to start walking. Both physically and mentally handicapped children sometimes look different and you should be prepared for this. They are often unco-ordinated and may move in a slightly jerky way.

Everyone involved in caring for handicapped children should help them to realise their abilities to the full. It would be doubly unfair if their disadvantages were exaggerated by lack of love and appreciation, lack of educational opportunity or enough knowledgeable care.

Physical handicaps

Encourage a child with a physical handicap to achieve independence and to help himself or herself. If you watch carefully, you will see when the child cannot manage and so know the right moment to give help.

Some children are born with physical handicaps, sometimes a disability may be the result of injury or illness. The degree of handicap varies from minor problems to the loss of movement or one or more senses. A child who is blind or deaf may learn more slowly and will certainly need skilled teaching.

Deafness

Deaf children often speak in strange flat voices, because they cannot hear other people or the sounds they make themselves. Partially deaf children can be helped by hearing aids. Totally deaf children need to be able to lip read so always face the child so he or she can see your lips. Speak slowly and clearly. You might find it useful to learn sign language if you care for a deaf child.

Testing hearing
A mother worried that her baby might be deaf should take him for a hearing test.

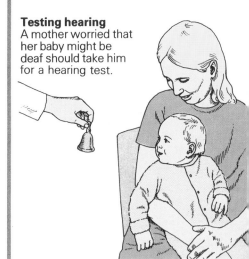

Blindness

Blind children usually like to touch you to get to know you. They often develop a very sharp sense of hearing and smell and can achieve a great measure of independence when experienced teachers show them how to find their way about. Blind children learn to read and write Braille, a system of raised dots on paper.

Children with limited movement

Some of these children may use wheelchairs and become expert at getting around. They may be able to transfer to a wheelchair without help. If not, you will need to work with a helper to get a child into a wheelchair if he or she is heavy. You can use the bed-to-chair lift described on page 21. Make sure the wheelchair brake is on first and always put the brake on if you have to leave the chair unattended. A wheelchair or walking aid appropriate for the child will be provided or recommended by the hospital or local social services.

When you are manoeuvring the chair up or down a kerb, take care to stay in control. Most chairs have a tipping lever to help you tilt them back. Make sure that both back or both front wheels touch the ground at the same time. Some children may have electric wheelchairs which they operate by pressing on a small knob. The chairs travel at a walking pace and give a child more independence. See that a child in a wheelchair is warmly enough dressed and that any coverings cannot get caught in the wheel spokes.

Occasionally a child may need his or her legs supporting with calipers (leg irons). With calipers on a child can usually walk quite well. Artificial limbs

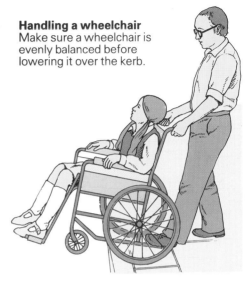

Handling a wheelchair
Make sure a wheelchair is evenly balanced before lowering it over the kerb.

are devices which substitute for a child's own limbs. The child will have been taught how to use the limb and may just need your assistance in putting it on or removing it.

Everyday care

Physically handicapped children may need extra help with dressing. Always put a disabled limb into a piece of clothing first. Remember to pull the clothes and not the child (see pages 34–35 for information on dressing and undressing). Offer help with meals as shown on page 56. Always find out first how much the child can do alone before you step in and do something for him or her.

Be patient with a child who has a speech difficulty or who is learning to lip read. The response will come if you give the child time and encouragement.

Help the child to be accepted by other children, explaining that, "his legs won't work properly," or, "she will hear you if you speak clearly".

Mental handicaps

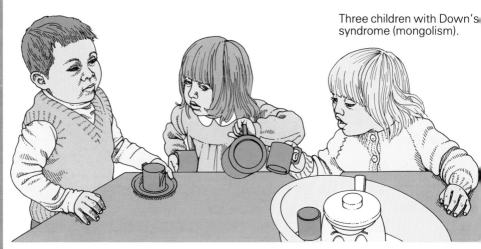

Three children with Down's syndrome (mongolism).

Sometimes a baby's brain does not develop normally or it may be damaged by injury or illness. The severity of the resulting handicap varies a great deal. The child will probably be slow to learn and is often described as having a mental age which is younger than his or her real age.

Patient teaching with a great deal of individual attention is necessary. Lessons may need to be repeated before the child absorbs any information or masters simple tasks like feeding or dressing.

Pressures on the family

Most mentally handicapped children are loving and respond warmly to affection. However, they can be very demanding because they need more care than the average child. The emotional pressure, practical and financial difficulties felt by the parents may be a great strain. They should seek advice from medical professionals and help from the Social Services Department right from the beginning. District nurses or special therapists may already be involved in looking after the child but any extra help you can offer will be welcomed by the parents.

Everyday care

Anyone caring for these children needs great powers of love and patience and must be alert. The mentally handicapped child may not understand the dangers involved in crossing roads of plugging in a kettle. Protect the child from injury but do not shelter him or her so much that you restrict life more than necessary. If you are helping to care for a mentally handicapped child, find out about any specially supervised swimming or riding lessons in the area. The child might find a great deal of pleasure in physical activities like these, in play with other children of similar ability, in music or in helping with basic household tasks.

You may need to guide the child's play because he or she might not have much curiosity to explore and learn from the environment. Provide simple toys. With encouragement the child will reach his or her full potential.

Aids in nursing

Some gadgets can greatly increase the independence of someone who is ill or handicapped by reducing the effort involved in simple essential tasks like getting washed and dressed. These aids are widely available but some of them are expensive. The local social services or hospital will often provide equipment such as walking aids or wheelchairs. Appropriate aids might make a really worthwhile improvement in the quality of life of anyone who is very elderly, arthritic, incontinent or with limited movement.

Mobility aids

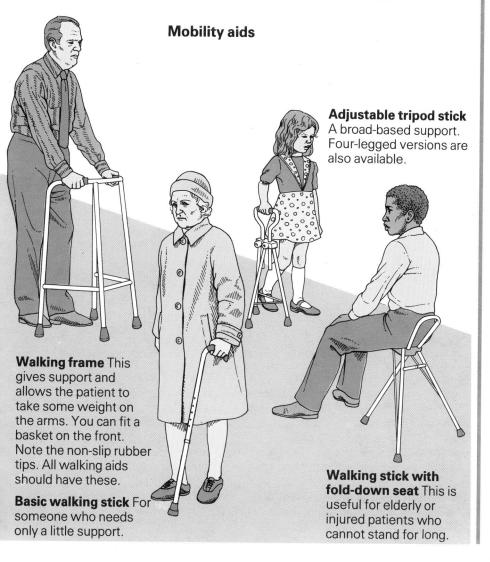

Adjustable tripod stick A broad-based support. Four-legged versions are also available.

Walking frame This gives support and allows the patient to take some weight on the arms. You can fit a basket on the front. Note the non-slip rubber tips. All walking aids should have these.

Basic walking stick For someone who needs only a little support.

Walking stick with fold-down seat This is useful for elderly or injured patients who cannot stand for long.

Aids for dressing

The aids shown here are some of the ones which are most useful to anyone with a weak grip or who cannot bend or stretch. The elderly, stroke patients and people with arthritis or rheumatism will find such aids enable them to get dressed much more easily and to remain fairly independent.

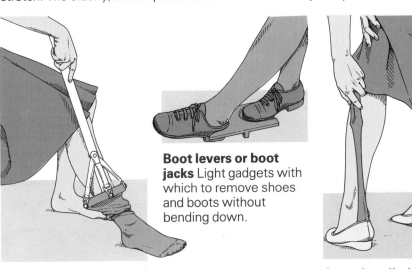

Boot levers or boot jacks Light gadgets with which to remove shoes and boots without bending down.

Stocking aid This kind clips on to the stocking, holding it open to pull up.

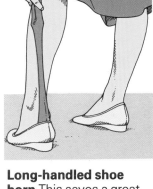

Long-handled shoe horn This saves a great deal of bending.

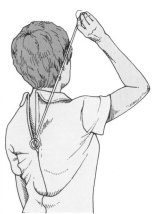

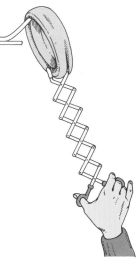

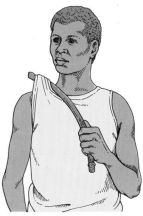

Trouble with zips Problems can be avoided by threading a long piece of string through the zip.

Lazy tongs One of several similar light and inexpensive gadgets which save on reaching.

Dressing stick This is a coat-hanger with a rubber thimble on the end to stop fabric slipping.

Bathroom aids

With these aids the bathroom can be made a great deal safer and more convenient for anyone who is very elderly or disabled.

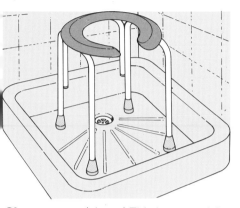

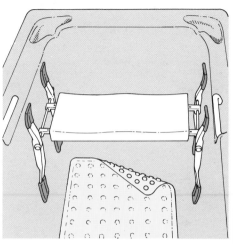

Shower seat (above) This is essential for the elderly or those who cannot stand for long.

Bath seat and non-slip mat A seat provides essential support for anyone who cannot get down to the bottom of the bath. The mat is held in place by suction caps.

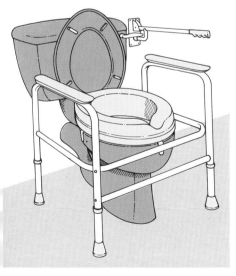

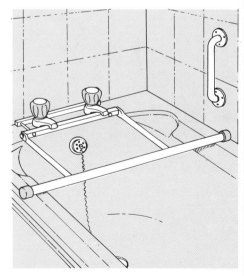

Lavatory frame and raised seat These enable patients with limited muscle power to lever themselves up or down or from a wheelchair.

Handrails There are many different kinds of handrail which can be fitted to the bath, or round the taps or to the wall, making it easier to get in or out.

Preventing accidents

Every year far more people are injured in accidents at home than on the roads. Accidents are the commonest cause of death among toddlers and older children. Yet many potential household hazards can be avoided by careful planning of the home and by common sense in the way you live.

Tidiness is common sense. If possessions are left lying around on the staircase or in the passages, or if boots are left on the floor by the entrance, someone could easily trip and fall. Be particularly careful when you are in a hurry, at times of stress such as moving house or when someone is ill. These are the times when accidents are most likely to occur.

If you have the opportunity to plan the furniture and fittings in your home, bear in mind the safety considerations and labour-saving devices shown on the following pages. Develop good safety habits, particularly when there are children or elderly people around. The common-sense caution which leads you to put medicines away and cover hot water bottles should be extended to other activities and all parts of the house. Do not carry pills in handbags when inquisitive children are around, they could be fatal.

It is a good idea to take a first aid course so that if an accident does occur, you will be able to react quickly and efficiently.

Children and accidents

You will not be able to prevent all minor accidents. The occasional cut or graze will happen despite your efforts. However, you can prevent serious accidents to children if you always take care to:
● teach a healthy respect for electricity by switching off the supply and unplugging appliances. Put blank plugs in empty sockets, especially if they are near the floor
● never leave plastic bags around in reach of a child who might put it over his or her head and suffocate
● put poisons such as bleach, ammonia and paint stripper out of reach, preferably locked away
● never leave a hot teapot or any hot container near the edge of a surface and never carry hot liquid when you are holding a baby
● teach a child about road safety and how to swim so that he or she can explore outside the home more safely
● keep small children within your sight or hearing
● keep possible hiding places locked; a child might be able to get into cupboards or the freezer and the door could close accidentally.

Old people

Most elderly people could avoid some common hazards in their home by simple safeguards like these:
● keep a stand by the front door to hold umbrellas and any walking aids when they are not in use
● put a chair on the landing and in passages if there is enough room so that an elderly person can rest if he or she becomes breathless
● fit a security chain and spy hole to the front door so that it is possible to check who visitors are before opening the door
● always check that any gas appliances have been turned off after use, as the elderly person's sense of smell may not be good. If it is very bad, suggest using electricity instead.

The entrance hall

Have light switches in convenient places, ideally one by the front door and one by the door of the main room leading off the entrance hall or by the stairs.

Safety locks on the door ensure that a toddler cannot go out on the road.

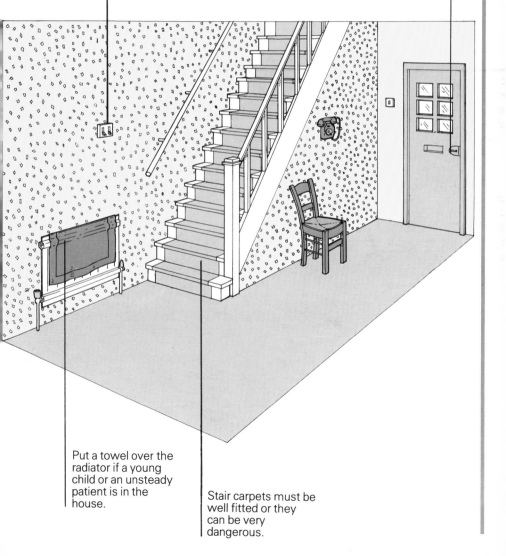

Put a towel over the radiator if a young child or an unsteady patient is in the house.

Stair carpets must be well fitted or they can be very dangerous.

Kitchen safety

Remember how curious children are and turn pan handles so that they do not stick out into the room. Leave floors and surfaces uncluttered, wiping up any spills as they happen. Do not have cloths hanging over the edge of the table. A toddler could easily pull a table cloth and anything on it down on to himself or herself.

Put matches away and hang any tea towels well away from the stove in case of fire. Always use any oven glove when removing hot dishes from the oven. Do not reach across a hot burner or ring, you could burn yourself or knock something off the cooker.

Aids in the kitchen

A long-handled dustpan and brush, right, will save any bending.

A steady trolley, below, makes it unnecessary to carry heavy dishes and acts as a walking aid.

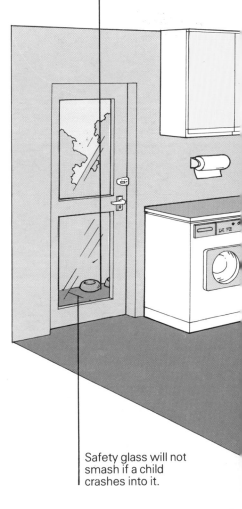

Put any pets' bowls outside or off the floor so a child cannot poke fingers into them.

Safety glass will not smash if a child crashes into it.

Fit childproof locks to the washing machine and dishwasher

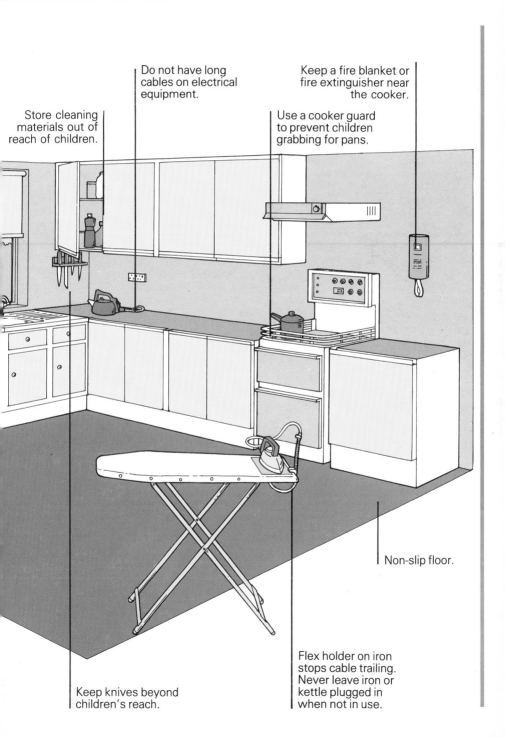

Do not have long cables on electrical equipment.

Keep a fire blanket or fire extinguisher near the cooker.

Store cleaning materials out of reach of children.

Use a cooker guard to prevent children grabbing for pans.

Non-slip floor.

Keep knives beyond children's reach.

Flex holder on iron stops cable trailing. Never leave iron or kettle plugged in when not in use.

The living room

This is often the most comfortable room in the house but it too will have potential hazards which you should be aware of. Make sure that all electrical equipment such as lamps, heaters, television and stereo is correctly wired. Most plugs are sold with instructions on how to fit them and these must be followed exactly. Run flexes round the walls if they are at floor level and gather up any spare cable, holding it neatly with a wire tie.

If you have an open fire and there are children in the house, use a fixed guard with a fine spark-proof mesh. Gas and electric heaters should also be fitted with secure guards. Paraffin heaters are dangerous and should not be used.

Put alcohol away, preferably in a locked cupboard. Never leave a hot or alcoholic drink within reach of children, it could burn them or make them ill. You should also put sewing materials away when there are children around. Sharp needles and scissors can be really dangerous when a toddler is at the stage of putting everything into his or her mouth. For the same reason, put away fire lighters, cigarettes, lighters and matches and do not keep breakable objects on low surfaces.

Floors and doors

Any rugs should have non-slip backing if they are on a wooden foor. Do not let toddlers run around in socks, they are more likely to skid and fall. Swing doors are frequently a cause of minor accidents when old people or toddlers are in the house. Their co-ordination is not good enough to avoid pinched fingers. Secure a swing door in an open position or replace it with a standard door which poses no danger.

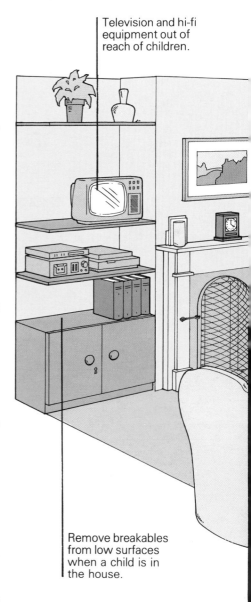

Television and hi-fi equipment out of reach of children.

Remove breakables from low surfaces when a child is in the house.

Fine mesh fireguard fixed to wall.

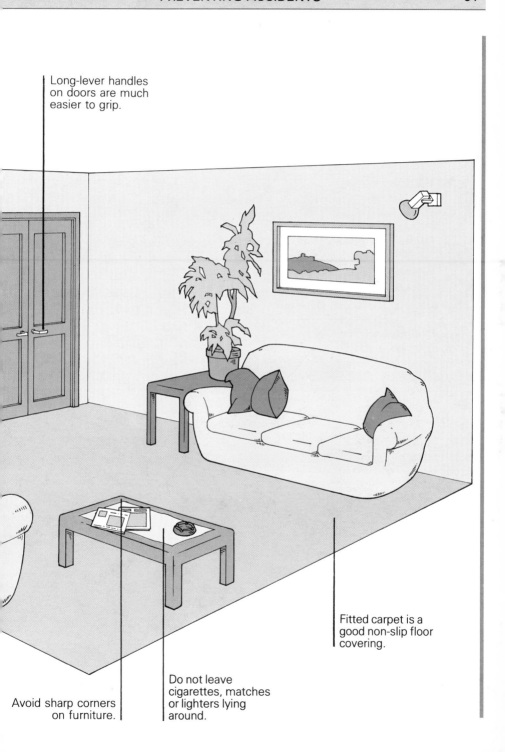

Long-lever handles on doors are much easier to grip.

Fitted carpet is a good non-slip floor covering.

Avoid sharp corners on furniture.

Do not leave cigarettes, matches or lighters lying around.

Stairs and windows

These are obvious danger areas, particularly for children, elderly people and anyone in a hurry. Children have to learn that climbing can be dangerous and silly as well as fun. Try to protect them from bad falls which could result in serious injuries.

Stairs

Carpets on staircases must be properly fitted so that they do not slip. Any worn patches should be removed or repaired so that they do not cause someone to trip. Always move clutter off the staircase, it could cause a nasty fall. Banisters should be closely spaced and vertical so a child cannot climb on them. Board up horizontal banisters. Stair rails must be well fixed, preferably on both sides to steady an old person. When children are young, fit safety gates to the stairs both top and bottom. They can easily be removed later. Make sure there is good light over the stairs.

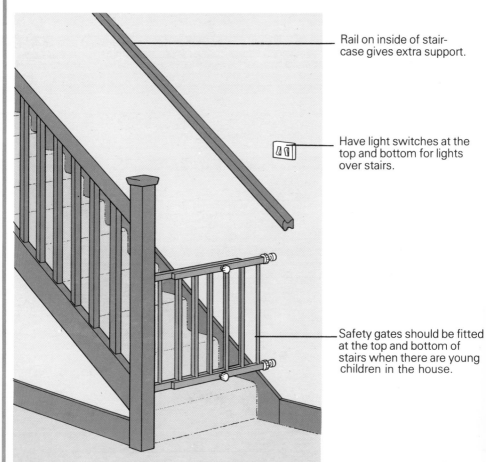

Rail on inside of staircase gives extra support.

Have light switches at the top and bottom for lights over stairs.

Safety gates should be fitted at the top and bottom of stairs when there are young children in the house.

Windows

These can be very dangerous when a toddler starts exploring. A small child does not have good balance and could easily fall out of a high unprotected window. Do not keep chairs or anything a child might climb on under a window. It is a good idea to put safety catches on all upstairs windows; there are many different kinds available. If there is a large expanse of glass in the child's bedroom, consider a grille or bars.

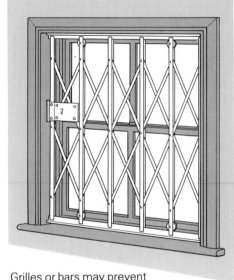

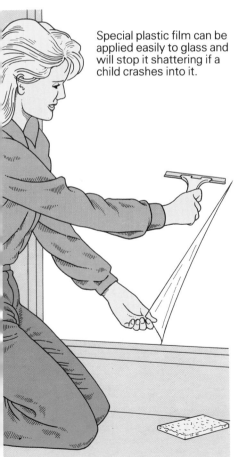

Special plastic film can be applied easily to glass and will stop it shattering if a child crashes into it.

Grilles or bars may prevent accidents but should be removable in case of fire.

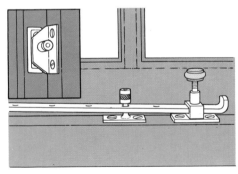

Common kinds of window catch. Keep the keys out of child's reach.

Index

A

Accident prevention 86–93
Adhesive dressings 63, 65
Aids, nursing 83
Armpit, taking temperature in 49
Arms
  bandages 66
  slings 68–9
Artificial limbs 81

B

Babies
  bathing 9, 33
  bedrooms 10–11
  brain damage 80, 82
  breathing rate 49
  clothes 36–7
  cots 9, 13
  dressing and undressing 36–7
  equipment 9
  feeding 58–61
  gastroenteritis 74
  immunisation 75
  nappies 42–4
  preparation for 9
  stools 38, 39
  weaning 61
Back problems, comfort in bed 24
Backrests 24
Bacteria 8, 64, 72
Bandages 62–3, 66–9
Barrier cream 27
Bath mats 85
Bath seats 29, 85
Bathing 28–9
  aids 85
  babies 9, 33
  bed baths 30
Bathrooms 29
  aids 85
Bed baths 30
Bed boards 24
Bed cradles 24
Bed sores, see pressure sores
Bed-wetting 41, 45, 77
Bedding 13
Bedpans 40, 41
Bedrooms
  adaptation 8
  for babies 10–11
  preparation 6–7

Beds 6
  bedding 13
  bed-ridden patients 12
  comfort in 24–7
  making 14–17
  moving patients alone 22–3
  moving patients in 18–19
  moving patients out of 21
  patient's position in 26
  stripping 14
  turning patients 20
  warmth in 25
Bending, elderly 78
Bladder
  incontinence 40–1
  learning control of 45
Blankets 13, 25
Blindness 80, 81
  feeding blind patients 56
Boot levers 84
Bottle-feeding, babies 60–1
Bowel
  incontinence 41
  learning control of 45
Brain damage 80, 82
Breast-feeding 58, 59
Breathing rate 49

C

Calipers 81
Carbohydrates 54
Carry-cots 9
Chairs, moving patient onto 21
Chickenpox 73
Children
  accident prevention 86
  bowel and bladder control 45
  cleaning teeth 32
  diet 52
  giving medicine to 50
  handicapped 80–2
  immunisation 75
  infectious diseases 72–5
  injuries 64, 65
  leaving hospital 77
  occupying in bed 47
  special diets 57
Chiropodists 31
Cleanliness 8
  personal 28–33
Clothes 34–5
  baby's 36–7
  dressing aids 35, 84
  elderly 78
Cold compresses 70, 71
Cold water packs 70
Colic 58
Comfort in bed 24–7
Commodes 6, 40

Compresses, cold 70, 71
Constipation 39, 53
Convenience foods 53
Corners, mitred 14
Cots 9, 13
Crockery 53
Cutlery 53
Cuts and grazes 64

D

Daily routines 46–61
Damp washing, hair 31
Deafness 80
Dehydration 39
Dentures, cleaning 32
Diabetes 49, 57
Diarrhoea 38, 39, 61, 74
Diet 52–7
  breast-feeding 59
  elderly 78
  infectious diseases 74
  roughage 41, 54
  special diets 57
Disease, infectious 72–5
Disposable nappies 42, 43
Disposable thermometers 47
Doors, safety 90
Drawsheets 14, 17
Dressing 34–5
  aids 35, 84
  babies 36–7
  handicapped children 81
Dressings 62–3, 65
Dry shampooing 31
Duvets 13

E

Elderly
  accident prevention 86
  nursing 78–9
Electricity, safety 86
Elimination 38–45
Entrance halls, safety 87
Excretions 38–45
Exercise, for elderly 78, 79

F

Face, washing 29
Faeces 39
  incontinence 40, 41
Fats, in diet 54
Feeding babies 58–61
Feeding cups 53
Feet, bandages 67
Feverish patients 28–9

Fibre, dietary 41, 54
Fingernails, care of 31
Floors, safety 90
Flu 73
Fluid-only diet 57
Food see diet
Footrests 24
Fresh air 8, 10

G

Gastroenteritis 73, 74
German measles 73, 74, 75
Germs 8, 64, 72
Grazes 64

H

Hair care 31
Handicapped children 80–2
Handrails 85
Hands, washing 29
Hearing tests 80
Heating
  baby's room 10
  for elderly 78
  patient's room 25
  safety 90
High chairs 9
Home, accident prevention
  86–93
Hospital, leaving 77
Hot poultices 70, 71
Hot water bottles 25
Hygiene 8, 38, 75
  personal 28–33
Hypothermia 47, 48, 78

I

Ice packs 70
Immunisation 75
Immunity 75
Incontinence 40–1
Incontinence aids 40
Incontinence pads 14, 17
Incubation period 72, 73, 75
Infectious diseases 72–5
Inflammation 70–1
Influenza 73
Inhalation, medicine 51
Injections 49
  immunisation 75
Injuries 62–71
Insomnia 78–9
Insulin injections 49
Iron, in diet 55

K

Kaolin poultices 70, 71
Kitchens, accident prevention
  88–9
Knots, reef 68–9

L

Lavatory frames 85
Lazy tongs 84
Lifting, by elderly 79
Lifting patients 18–19
Light diets 57
Liquid medicines 50
Living rooms, safety 90–1
Low-calorie diets 57

M

Massage, to prevent pressure
  sores, 27
Mattresses, cot 9
Meals 52–7
  see also diet
Measles 73, 75
Medicines 49
  by mouth 50
  inhalation 51
  medicine cupboard 62–3
  safety 8, 49, 86
Menstruation 38
Mental handicaps 80, 82
Milk
  bottle-feeding 60
  breast-feeding 59
  mineral salts, in diet 55
Mitred corners, sheets 14
Mobility aids 83
Mouth
  care of 32
  taking temperature in 47,
    48–9
Mouthwashes 32
Mumps 73, 74
Muslin nappy liners 42

N

Nails, care of 31
Nappies 42–4
Nappy liners 42
Nappy rash 44
Nelson's inhaler 51
Nightdresses 35
Nursing aids 83

O

Observations 46–7
Orthopaedic bed boards 24
Overweight 57

P

Patients
  beds 12–17
  clothes 34–5
  comfort in bed 24–7
  daily routines 46–61
  diet 52–7
  dressing and undressing
    34–5
  elderly 78–9
  elimination 38–45
  infectious diseases 72–5
  injuries 62–71
  leaving hospital 77
  moving 18–23
  observation 46–7
  occupying in bed 47
  personal care 28–45
  position in bed 26
  preparation for 6–8
Periods, monthly 38
Personal care 28–45
Perspiration 28
Physical handicaps 80–1
Pillows 24, 26
  triangular-shaped 24
Pills 50
Plastic pants 44
Plastic sheets 14
Playpens 10
Potty training 45
Poultices 70, 71
Powders, medicinal 50
Pressure sores 12, 20, 27
Prostate gland 41
Protein 54
Pulse 46, 48–9

R

Rashes 74
Records 46
Reef knots 68–9
Roller bandages 63, 66–7
Roughage 41, 54

S

Safety 8
  accident prevention 86–93
  baby's room 10
  medicines 8, 49, 86
Safety pins, nappies 42
Saliva 32
Sheepskin pads 24, 27
Sheets 13
  bedmaking 14–17
  drawsheets 14, 17
  mitred corners 14
  plastic 14
Shoe horns 84
Shower seats 29, 85
Showers 29
Sleeplessness 78–9
Slings 68–9
Smoking, safety 8
Sores, pressure 12, 20, 27
Special nursing 76–85
Specimens 38
Sponging down 29, 74
Sputum 38
Stairs, safety 92
Steam inhalation 51
Sterile dressings 63, 65
Sterilising
  feeding equipment 61–2
  nappies 44
Stocking aids 84
Stools 38, 39
Stress incontinence 40–1
Stretch suits, babies 36
Strip thermometers 47
Stripping a bed 14

T

Tablets 50
Teats, bottle-feeding 60
Teeth
  cleaning 32
  decay 32
  eating without 56
Temperature 28–9
  hypothermia 47, 48, 78
  lowering 29, 74
  taking 46, 47–9
Terry towelling nappies 42–3
Thermometers 47
Toenails, care of 31
Toilet training 45
Triangular bandages 63, 68
Tripod sticks 83
Trousers, putting on 34

U

Undressing 34–5
  babies 37
Urinals 40, 41
Urine 38
  incontinence 40–1

V

Ventilation 8, 10
Vitamins 55
Vomiting 38, 39

W

Walking frames 83
Walking sticks 83
Warmth, in bed 25
Washing 28–9
  aids 85
  bed baths 30
  hair 31
  nappies 44
Water, in diet 54
Weaning 61
Wheelchairs 81, 83
Whooping cough 73, 75
Wind 58
Windows, safety 10, 93
Wounds, care of 64–5
  inflammation 70–1

Z

Zinc and castor oil cream 44
Zips, dressing aids 84

Acknowledgments

Project editor Jemima Dunne
Editor Katie Cohen

Designers Carole Ash, Julia Harris

Managing editor Daphne Razazan
Art editor Anne-Marie Bulat

Photography Paul Fletcher

Typesetting Cambrian Typesetters